The Success Habits of Weight-Loss Surgery Patients

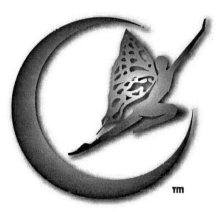

COLLEEN M. COOK

Printed in the United States of America
Third Printing 2010

Published by Bariatric Support Centers International
9257 South Redwood Road, Suite B, West Jordan, Utah 84088
www.bariatricsupportcenter.com

IBSN 0-9740179-7-3

To those early bariatric patients and professionals whose willingness to share their successes and failures have taught us all the importance of these principles.

To Roger, Craig, Chris & Miranda Cook for their belief in me, their encouragement and their many sacrifices on behalf of this work.

To Janean Hall, Tammy Bartz, Dana Schroeder, Sue Lassetter and the BSCI staff members for their belief in the importance of this work, their commitment to its future development, and their constant and consistent dedication to our mission.

To Ken Miller for his strength, his far reaching vision and his unwavering commitment to excellence.

What Bariatric Patients and Professionals are saying:

""The Success Habits™ principles and the programs Colleen uses to teach them are helping patients ensure their long-term success following weight-loss surgery. She has educated and motivated both my patients and my support group leaders."

    -MAL Fobi, M.D., F.A.C.S.
    Hawaiian Gardens, CA

"Colleen's presentation moved our investigators and our patients, both. I thank Colleen for the dedication she has manifested in guiding patients and bariatric surgical programs"

    - Robert T. Marema, M.D., F.A.C.S.
    Ft. Lauderdale, FL

"Colleen's sharing of her personal insight into the disease of morbid obesity and its recovery through surgery was inspirational to our group."

    - J K Champion, M.D., F.A.C.S.
    Atlanta, GA

"I liked this book so much I decided to buy another one for a friend. Boy is she in for a treat! This is by far the very best material written for WLS patients"

    - D. Klee, WLS Patient 2004

"I have been very pleased with the Back On Track Program and the level of support I have received. It's value to me has been immeasurable."

    - Pam Eppel, WLS Patient 1993

"Colleen Cook is both an exceptional student and instructor. She possesses the ability to synthesize complex information and then to distill and share it, helping others to understand in a motivational format. She wants everyone to succeed with the foundation of knowledge which will facilitate that success. I have thoroughly enjoyed watching her succeed with her own life while nurturing others to follow her fine example."

    - Sherman C. Smith, M.D., F.A.C.S.
     Salt Lake City, UT

"I would highly recommend BSCI's Support Group Leader training course to anyone that facilitates a support group or works with bariatric patients. The classes were fun and educational. We learned how to motivate and encourage others. The importance of accountability and commitments was demonstrated through fun interactive games and activities."

    - Carolyn Williams, FNP,
     Mayo Clinic, Scottsdale, AZ

"We appreciate BSCI so much for providing a reliable source of education and support for patients and professionals alike. The training and services they make available (always with a smile!) have raised the role of the support giver to a new level. As this community continues to expand rapidly, what they do becomes increasingly important."

    - Tom Kinder, President & CEO
    - J. Jacques, ND, Chief Science Officer
     Bariatric Advantage

CONTENTS

PREFACE

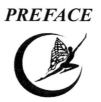

It is with great pleasure that we provide you with this 2nd Edition of The Success Habits of Weight-loss Surgery Patients. It has been four years since its first publication and we are happy to say that the principles taught here continue to be a standard for success throughout the bariatric community.

The Success Habits™ Principles are now taught in hundreds of bariatric support groups each month and are recommended by many Bariatric Centers of Excellence, surgeons and bariatric health professionals. They provide structure, clarity and simplicity for weight loss surgery patients as they reach and maintain a healthy weight.

Once again, we have consulted with respected bariatric professionals who have provided updates, clarification, and validation of these key lifetime principles.

You will find in this new edition a variety of real-life experiences from Gastric Bypass, LapBand®, Duodenal Switch, & Vertical Sleeve Gastrectomy weight-loss surgery patients. Each one has found success through the surgical treatment of their choice and by making the Success Habits an integral part of their lives.

Foreword

The caption on the poster read, "A Great Solution Doesn't Have To Be Complicated." I mounted it on the wall in my office where it held a place of honor for over ten years. Whenever I sat back in my chair and contemplated how to solve a particularly difficult problem, its message served as a constant yardstick by which I measured the value of each new idea or potential solution to an engineering obstacle I was trying to overcome. In my work as a mechanical engineer in the research department of a major US explosives company, I designed equipment that was used to make explosives, or package them, or deliver them into boreholes.

My work took me to the far corners of the earth where the equipment I designed was used to advance mining and excavation technology in ways that had never been accomplished before. My control and delivery systems were used when the world's first large single-shot blast of 600,000 pounds of explosives was detonated in an underground mine in Sudbury, Ontario, Canada. My equipment helped level the island where the new Hong Kong Airport was built. During the course of my career as a research engineer in the explosives industry, I was awarded four United States patents for new and innovative methods of solving some very difficult technical problems. Throughout my 15-year career in that industry, I was constantly guided by the principle that was so perfectly illustrated on that poster.

The poster was printed by the Grumman Aircraft Corporation, makers of world-class fighter jets, who thought its message to be so important they paid for an ad in one of the engineering trade magazines I received each month. They offered to send engineers a free, full-size copy of the poster and they didn't care whether I worked in the aircraft industry or not. The first time I saw it I knew I had to have one of those posters! You see, in the engineering world, it's relatively easy to add another feature to your design, making it a little more complex than it was, whenever a problem is discovered in operation. This tendency to ADD complexity to solve problems results in products that may work fairly well when they're new, but they're much more difficult to maintain because more parts mean more opportunities for the product to breakdown and fail. And, more complexity means that its operator or maintenance person must be more highly educated and intelligent than would be necessary if a simpler design were used to solve the same problem.

Now, there's a dilemma! And a mental paradox. It requires MUCH more work and effort to simplify a design, (or anything else for that matter), than it does to make it more complex. So, unless an engineer is constantly on guard to prevent complexities from creeping into his designs, they will be added here and there until his final product is too complex for the average person to use.

Regardless of how well your solution to someone's problem might be, if it's too complex or difficult for them to use in real situations, they will set it aside and go back to their old method of "solving" their problem, even if that way is less efficient than your "new and improved" solution.

In my early days as an engineer, I learned this lesson the hard way. I designed equipment without taking the time to interview the final users of that equipment. I stupidly thought that I was "more qualified", through my education and training, than they were and that my solutions would automatically be better than theirs because I was specially trained to solve these kinds of problems. Boy, was I wrong. I quickly learned that NO ONE knows more about the problems faced by the operator than the operator does; and NO ONE knows more about the problems faced by the maintenance person than the maintenance person does.

After I developed a few "solutions" to their problems, had installed those "solutions" and watched them work successfully while I was standing there directly supervising them, I'd move on to my next project. Later when I returned from my office to the production floor (where the real-world determines what works and what doesn't), there I would find my solution to their problem sitting in a corner-cast aside while they were busily doing their best to keep up with production schedules using their old way of doing things. Then I began to learn what the real problems were that the real-world operators faced. Real-world operators are experienced enough to know it's a total waste of their time to try to tell an "expert" what their real needs are and why the expert's solution will not work in their situation. Generally, the expert knows too much for them to be able to help him.

Thankfully, after a couple of sad experiences, I learned to interview the real-world operators and maintenance people BEFORE I started developing "new and improved" solutions for their problems. Only then did my "solutions" truly excel. The combination of their real-world experience and my technical training, working together, produced solutions that were simple and effective; AND they were easy to operate and maintain. Those solutions became part of their everyday world and were never cast aside. They survived and were used because they actually improved the lives of the people who used them.

And so it is with this book. Colleen Cook, a gastric bypass patient since 1995, has taken the real-world experiences of thousands of weight-loss surgery patients and condensed them into the principles you'll find in this book. These principles are time and people tested. They work regardless of the particular type of weight-loss surgery you may have had. They are universal truths that have been proven by the successes and failures of thousands of individuals. Those WLS patients who live by these principles successfully lose their excess weight, and are able to control their weight thereafter. WLS patients who have not understood these principles-or have chosen to ignore them-and have regained much of their former weight, have been able to turn around, get back on track, lose significant amounts of weight, and then keep it off by adopting these same principles.

During the course of my association with Colleen, and our joint efforts to create and expand Bariatric Support Centers International, we've heard from many people who say something like this, "I don't follow [this Success Habit™ principle] and I'm doing just fine. I'm down to a size [whatever] and I've kept my weight off for [number of months]. I have a new life and I don't have to live all of the Success Habits™ principles." Usually, these people are less than two years post-op and the realities of long-term maintenance haven't really hit them yet.

Yes, there are those who may be able to ignore one or two of the lesser Success Habits™ principles and can still maintain their weight-loss. But for every single person who can do this, there are 100 who can't, and, like finding out who's an alcoholic and who's not, it's impossible to tell which person you really are until it's too late to go back and develop the Success Habits when it's easiest to change–during the first year post-op. My advice to those of you who are considering weight-loss surgery, and those of you who have had weight-loss surgery and want to make sure that THIS time you're going to achieve your FINAL SUCCESS and maintain your desired weight for the rest of your life . . . learn the Success Habits™ principles and live them. If you do, you'll achieve that final success.

You may have noticed that we call them Success Habits™ PRINCIPLES, not rules. When you learn to understand them correctly, they will be guiding principles by which you can make decisions in thousands of different situations and circumstances. In this fast-paced world where we live, things are constantly changing; it's impossible to make up rules fast enough to cover all of the situations you'll encounter. When we are subjected to rules, we feel deprived. When we live by principles, we feel guided and directed by our own best choices. When we live rule-based lives, we spend our time and emotional efforts looking for loopholes that will allow us to pretend its okay for us to do something that we know is questionable. When we live our lives by the guidance of principles, WE become the ultimate judge of whether or not we are keeping the principles we've chosen to guide our decisions. We feel like slaves to rules, but living a principle-centered life sets us free to become our highest and best self.

So . . . what does all of this talk about designing for simplicity and living by principles have to do with The Success Habits™ of Weight-Loss Surgery Patients? Just this... Colleen could have written a highly technical book on the science behind these Success Habits™ principles, and she could have written a much longer book that expressed these ideas from the point of view of an "expert" who is here to impress you with how smart she is. Impressing you with the complexities of weight-loss surgery and its technical effects on your body was not her goal. Colleen has focused first and foremost on simplifying these principles so they can be understood and implemented in the lives of people from all walks of life. After all, the real measure of a solution's value is not how complex it looks or sounds; the real measure is how well it actually works. It takes much more work and effort to create an elegant, simple solution for a difficult problem than it does to create a solution that is so complex and hard to use that it is cast aside by the user.

May you be wise enough to recognize the value of time-tested, simple truths; and may they lead to your own personal Final Success.

Oh, by the way, speaking of simple, elegant solutions to long term problems... the picture on the poster with the caption that read, "A Great Solution Doesn't Have To Be Complicated", was a close-up photograph of a simple paper clip.

Kenneth A. Miller, 2001-2006 President
Bariatric Support Centers International

INTRODUCTION

No one was expecting it. But there it was. An idea that would profoundly affect hundreds of thousands of weight-loss surgery patients for years to come. As is often the case, the solution for the future was found by analyzing the past.

A weight-loss surgery patient from 1995 with a background in speaking and facilitating, I had accepted a position as director of the Center for the Surgical Treatment of Obesity for St. Mark's Hospital in Salt Lake City, Utah, to coordinate and improve the hospital's bariatric support group program. I was attending a regularly scheduled early-morning meeting with three bariatric surgeons. Among them was a true pioneer in the field of bariatrics, Dr. Gerald Goodman. He and his partner, the late Dr. David K. Miller, had begun performing Roux-en-Y weight-loss surgery procedures in the late 1970s. Like Barbara Mandrell's song, "I Was Country When Country Wasn't Cool," these dedicated surgeons were doing bariatric surgery when bariatric surgery wasn't cool.

As the surgical treatment for obesity became more widely understood and accepted, hundreds of new surgeons throughout the country looked to them not only for their experience in surgical technique but for what they had that no one else did: thousands of long-term patients who had undergone weight-loss surgery 10, 15, and even 20 years prior. Everyone, both professionals and patients, asked, "How are they doing? Are they healthy? Have they maintained their weight loss over time?"

I recall in great detail the discussion at that meeting. Perplexed, Dr. Charles B. Edwards posed the question, "Why can one patient who has this surgical procedure maintain weight loss year after year, and another patient, who has the identical procedure, lose substantial weight and then regain it?" We could all clearly see the powerful effect the answer to this question would have on the success of future patients.

Experience had taught that often the returning patients that had regained some weight had initially followed the dietary and behavioral guidelines they had been given. However, through the years, they returned to their old habits and had forsaken some or all of the new behaviors they had learned in the early years following their surgery. But why? Why were some able to comply, while others were not? Why did some learn that they alone were responsible for their success, while others expected the surgery to be the cure in and of itself.

It was apparent that faltering patients had a number of things in common. Dr. Edwards then suggested that perhaps we would also find some commonalities among the most successful patients. He suggested that if we could identify what the most successful patients had in common and couple that data with the knowledge of habits leading to failure, we could establish solid, well-defined guidelines for new patients to follow. It was determined that the most effective way to make these comparisons was through a formal survey. And so I began the original study of the habits of long-term weight-loss surgery patients.

I presented the results of the survey at the fifteenth annual meeting of the American Society for Bariatric Surgery in Orlando, Florida, on June 29, 1998. The report, "The Success Habits of Long-term Gastric Bypass Patients, by Cook and Edwards," was published in February 1999 in "Obesity Surgery Journal".

After the original study, I selected six habits common to the most successful patients. Through the years, I have continued to read and study, research and refine these key principles of weight loss and weight maintenance. I have come to believe, from my own experience as a patient and from the experiences of thousands of weight-loss surgery patients who have shared their stories with me, that they are important both individually and collectively.

In this book, I share the basic elements of these principles, my own experiences with them and what I have learned through study and from other patients and professionals in the bariatric field. These Success Habits™ principles are not new and they are not revolutionary, but I believe that compliance with them is essential to long-term weight-loss and good health following weight-loss surgery.

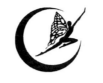

My New Beginning

I recall the early weeks following my surgery. There were so many thoughts and emotions to deal with. Thoughts like, "What have I done?" and "Will I ever feel normal again?" I hadn't told very many people about my decision prior to surgery. I have many nurse friends, and frankly, I didn't want to hear the horror stories that have circulated for so many years among medical professionals. So I didn't tell any of my friends until after the surgery had taken place.

I recall being in my hospital room and deciding to call one such friend, a nurse. When she answered the phone I told her where I was, that I was doing okay, and why I was there. I will never forget her immediate reply: "You are so lucky!"

Lucky? Having just had major surgery, I didn't feel so lucky. I felt quite unlucky, in fact. I had tried dozens of diets, pills, powders, exercise plans, behavior modification programs -the works- all without long-term success. While many struggle with thoughts that they have "cheated" or taken the easy way out, I have always regarded my decision to have weight-loss surgery as one of the best, most responsible decisions I have ever made. It wasn't luck, it wasn't cowardice; it was a good responsible decision for me, my health and my life.

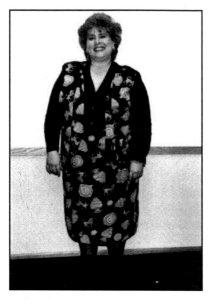

I quietly and secretly investigated weight-loss surgery in 1993. I had a personal consultation with a surgeon and knew that this was the answer for me. Unfortunately, my insurance would not cover it and paying cash was not a possibility at that time. So, I just kept it to myself and thought, "Someday, some way I will do this." Years passed and I reached my all-time heaviest weight of 250 pounds. At 5 feet, 2 inches, I was unhappy and unhealthy, but still my insurance wouldn't cover it.

On Thanksgiving weekend of 1995, my wonderful husband, knowing of my unhappiness and my deteriorating health, suggested that we take a second mortgage on our home and use the equity to pay cash for this surgery. Some of my friends were buying new cars and new furniture; I got a new body (and now I have the new car and the new furniture)! It was certainly a risk to undergo major surgery uninsured, but it was a risk we were willing to take. That decision has proven to be one of the best decisions I have ever made. It has been worth every penny of our investment; so much so that in December 2001, my husband, Roger, also had weight-loss surgery, and now he is much happier and healthier as well.

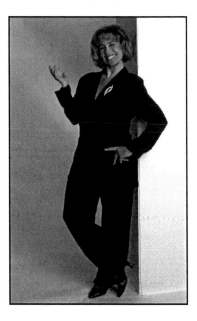

There were many changes to make during the first year as I adjusted to my new, post-surgery habits. Perhaps the most important change that I made was how I thought and felt about food. During the first several months, while my body was responding to the types and quantities of food I was eating, I decided that this was the time to learn to think differently about food. It proved to be an ideal time to learn to make this monumental transition. For example, I no longer saw a "sandwich," but rather a combination of separate food groups: protein (the meat and cheese), vegetables (the lettuce and tomato) and carbohydrates (the bread).

Several months later, after losing 50 pounds or so, I met a friend for lunch. A doughnut was part of the chili lunch special, and I decided that rather than waste it I would take it home to one of my teenagers. The server placed the doughnut in a little sack for me, and I was on my way with the doughnut on the passenger seat beside me. When I arrived home some 40 minutes later, as I pulled into the driveway, I was surprised when I noticed the doughnut! You see, prior to surgery, I would have been so aware of that doughnut on the seat, that it never would have made it out of the parking lot! I would have devoured it just as soon as my friend's car turned the corner! "Wow," I thought; a great change had occurred in how I related to food. I was not tempted by it; I was not consumed with thoughts of it. What a wonderful change!

I began to focus my attention on exercise and living a healthy lifestyle and redirected my energy from eating to shopping (also a potentially dangerous habit)! Dropping from a size 26 to an 8 in one year meant new clothes each week. I became quite a thrift store shopper and donor! (See Appendix A, Helpful People, Products, and Programs).

During the early months following your surgery, may I encourage you to use that golden time when your body is reacting in new ways to what and how much you eat, to change how you think and feel about food? Food will always be there, and will always be a temptation for you if you allow it to be. Change what food means to you. Learn that you must eat to live rather than live to eat.

Take full responsibility for and advantage of this most opportune time to make the Success Habits™ principles I am about to share with you part of the new you. Learn them, understand them, internalize them and turn your wonderful "New Beginning" into a lifetime of good health and happiness.

Success Habits™ *Principle 1*

Personal Accountability

*"I recognize that I alone am responsible for
my successes and my failures."*

To identify the most common habits or behaviors of the most successful, long-term weight-loss surgery patients, the most pressing questions I asked were about diet and exercise. From my own experience, I knew that I had to, somehow, gauge the level of personal commitment and responsibility of each of the patients we interviewed. I expected that if I simply asked, "Who is responsible for your success?" they would reply, "Well, I am, of course." Certainly, that does seem like the right answer, but how could we know for sure what, "I am responsible" meant to them? I had to come up with an indicator of just HOW they were assuming responsibility for their weight maintenance and WHAT they were doing regularly that was helping them stay in control and remain accountable for their weight every day. I came up with a few key questions, which will be discussed later in this chapter. Above all, I have always believed, that a person's ability to take responsibility for himself is a key to success in any arena.

Wherever you are right now, whatever your life looks like, whatever situation you find yourself in, I encourage you to live The First Success Habit Principle: Be personally accountable for the decisions you have made, take responsibility for your choices, and be honest with yourself. I believe that we are where we are because we have chosen to be so. Our lives must be serving us in some way or else we would have already made changes. Take responsibility for who, for what, and for where you are right now.

WHERE AM I?

I have enjoyed traveling as a professional speaker to places all over the country. I've been to some really wonderful cities, and places all over the United States, but more often than not I stay pretty close to home. I go a few hours east to Price, Utah, or a few hours south to St. George, Utah, and then a little east to Elko, Nevada, and other local hot spots.

On one occasion, I was asked to speak to a group in Pocatello, Idaho. Pocatello is just three hours due north of Salt Lake City; you just follow Interstate 15 north until you run into it. I was on my way in the early afternoon and was right on time. I had my little frozen bottle of water, some rock and roll going on the radio, and little munchies to eat. As I was driving along, I was being marriage counselor-of-the-week for a friend of mine on my cellular phone. As we finished our conversation, I hung up the phone and continued my drive. All of a sudden my Indian guide self, inside me, said, "Hmmm, if I am on my way from Salt Lake City straight north to Pocatello, Idaho at this hour of the after-noon the sun shouldn't be in my eyes." I thought, "Where am I? Where am I!" I was traveling seventy-five miles an hour, but I had no idea where I was or where I was heading. I thought, "Okay, what do I do? I have a map in the trunk, but the map is useless if I don't know where I am on the map." So I thought, "Well, I need to drive until I can figure out where I am. I need to find a sign. I didn't know whether to keep driving or go back; so I kept driving. I didn't see a sign, but I saw a truck stop. I pulled into the truck stop, where I found a Budweiser Beer guy. I thought he looked like a real nice, clean-cut guy, so I went over and asked, "Sir, where am I?"

And he said, "Well, you're on your way to Burley, Idaho."

"Oh, I need to be in Pocatello."

"Well, you're about an hour and a half out of your way. As we looked at the map he explained, "You need to go there and turn here." He explained it all.

Soon, I was back on my way just kind of shaking my head thinking to myself, "Wow, I need to pay a little more attention." I also thought it was kind of insightful that I did-n't know where I was, but I knew that it wasn't where I was supposed to be. I knew I was headed in the wrong direction.

A couple of years after that little incident, I was speaking at Utah State University in Logan, Utah. The conference went very well. I felt good about everything and I was driving home, straight south from Logan to Salt Lake City. As I was driving along, I thought, "It's a beautiful day." I looked about and, oh, it was wonderful. There were fluffy clouds, and blue skies, and butterflies, and chirping birds, and the sun was shining. I crossed rolling fields, past barns and cows . . . and more barns and more cows . . . and a few more barns . . . and a few more cows. And then I thought, "Now where am I?" And it hit me, I thought, "Oh man, I am off again!" I had learned from my Burley, Idaho experience that I needed to find a sign and figure out where I was. I drove a little further and saw a sign up ahead that said "Paradise, two miles." I thought, "Cool, I've never been to Paradise. I think I'll go to Paradise . . . and then I'll go home." As I drove into Paradise, I came upon a little country market; a corner store. As I pulled into the tiny parking lot, I saw another Budweiser Beer guy! So I said, "Sir, would you please tell me where I am supposed to be?"

He explained, "Oh yeah, you missed the fork as you were leaving Logan." He proceeded to give me directions back to the main highway and soon, I was on my way, back on track. On the way I thought, "I should know by now to pay attention when I drive, to take a map, and to not talk to strangers; all those kinds of things. But I learned some other very valuable things that day. I learned, first of all, that I would much rather live in Paradise than Burley, Idaho! The second thing I learned is that the Budweiser Beer guys always know where they are and where I'm supposed to be. And the third, and most important thing I learned is that my inner self, my inner child, my inner voice, whatever you want to call it; my "Indian guide," as I refer to it, is a pretty smart cookie. Sometimes I may be a little slow on the uptake, but I've learned it's important to rely on that inner compass. I didn't know where I was going or where I was at that moment, but I knew it simply felt wrong. It felt like I was not where I ought to be, could be, or should be.

I recognized that feeling from many years before, when I found myself at two hundred and fifty pounds working in a four by four foot cubicle in a call center, with my ear attached to the wire of a telephone. I remember distinctly, as I worked along one day, being overwhelmed by the thoughts, "Where am I? This is not where I belong! This is not where I'm supposed to be! This is not who I am! This isn't even what I look like!" It was that day I made the decision to take responsibility for where I was, and to do whatever it took to get where I needed to be. I had come to that point in my life where many of you have been or currently are. I have a very strong belief that, "Successful people do those things which unsuccessful people are not willing to do."

And so I made a very difficult and very drastic decision, as many of you have also made. I had weight-loss surgery in 1995. It was a difficult decision to have the surgical procedure, but I took that step. I took responsibility for where I was and how I got there. And I told myself the truth.

> "Successful people do those things which unsuccessful people are not willing to do."

Again, Success Habit Principle Number One is to take responsibility for who, for what, and for where you are right now and be honest with yourself; tell yourself the truth. Failure to do so will prohibit you from reaching the potential that is within you.

I believe that you are where you are right now because you have chosen to be so. Your life must be serving you in some way, or else you would have already made a change. Take a look at who you are, why you are, and where you are and take responsibility for how you arrived here.

Let me illustrate this concept by relating a story about two battleships at sea. Visibility was very poor, and the lookout called back to the captain on the ship and said, "There is a light on the starboard bow."

The captain asked, "Is it steady or moving astern?"

The reply came back from the lookout, "It is steady." This meant they were on a dangerous collision course.

And so the captain said, "Send a signal; send a signal that says, 'I command you to change your course twenty degrees'!"

The signal was sent and a reply came back, "You change course twenty degrees."

So the captain said, "Well, send a signal that says, 'I am a Captain. Change your course twenty degrees'."

The signal was sent and the reply came back, "I am a Seaman second class. You change course twenty degrees."

Now the captain was getting more upset as he thought, "It's getting more and more dangerous." He said, "Send a signal; send a very strong signal that says, 'We are a battleship. Change your course twenty degrees'!"

The signal was sent and again a reply came back; it simply said, "We are the lighthouse."

How often in our lives when we feel there is a need for change do we wait for someone else to make it?

Again, I encourage you to take responsibility. Recognize that you, and you alone, must be accountable for your long-term success following your weight loss surgery.

Personal Accountability is the first Success Habits™ principle. Each principle is important, but Personal Accountability is the most important factor contributing to optimum weight loss and long-term weight control. My hope is that you will study these concepts, understand them, remember them, internalize them and that you, too, will realize that your personal commitment to your own success is absolutely essential!

I have no doubt you've heard that surgical treatment for obesity provides you with a tool for your success. Bariatric surgery has the potential to serve you well your entire life, but only if you learn to use it properly. It is essential that you understand it is ONLY a tool. I, too, heard the words, "It is only a tool," but it was not until several years after my surgery that I came to a complete understanding of just what this means.

The basics of metabolism are and always have been very simple. It's all about the ratio of Calories-In versus Calories-Out. If you eat more than you expend in energy, you will gain weight. If you eat less that you expend, you will lose weight. That most basic truth will never change; not ever! Surgery does not cure obesity. Once again, it provides a tool which, if used properly, will help you gain and stay in control of that very basic principle: Calories-In versus Calories-Out. You and only you are responsible for what you eat, when you eat, and how much you eat.

Likewise, you are also responsible for your energy output; the level of activity you engage in, how often you exercise and how you control your energy expenditures each day. You and only you are responsible for making the lifetime commitment to these Success Habits™ principles. You and only you are responsible for your success!

There are probably other people in your life that would be willing to take this responsibility on FOR you; people who love you and would love to help you. You probably wish they could; you may resent them because they do not. But the reality is that no one else CAN. Willing or not, no one else can do this for you.

If you really want to change, and you're willing to put in a little bit of time and some concentrated thinking about why you do what you do, there is a process by which you can do so. For additional reading on this subject may I recommend BSCI's Exchanging Habits Book, by Kenneth A. Miller.

REGULAR WEIGHING

The most successful long-term weight-loss surgery patients are those who weigh themselves regularly. They each have a profound sense of personal responsibility for their success, regard their surgery as a tool, and are committed to always knowing where they are. They are keeping their weight in check.

A few years ago a patient attended one of my classes. After introducing herself, she expressed frustration. "I'm six years out of surgery, and suddenly I'm recognizing that I've regained 30 pounds!" she exclaimed. That works out to be an average of less than 1/2 pound per month. Not a significant weight gain day-to-day, but compound it over six years and it equals 30 pounds. It's easy for those ounces to add up to pounds over the years if we're not paying attention.

What a profound lesson this is for all of us. This woman was surprised to find that she had gained so much. The pounds sneaked up on her, ever so slowly, just a little bit at a time. Only half a pound per month, after month, after month, compounded into 5 pounds in one year. Reasonable, yes, but left unchecked and ignored, she gained another 5 pounds, and another 5 and another 5. Five pounds is nothing to lose. But 30 pounds becomes much more difficult. So, we can't just sit back and rest on our past weight-loss success without being vigilant about our current weight. But just how aware do we need to be? It's been my experience that weighing myself weekly is the best indicator of progress or the lack thereof. More frequently than once a week can become a bit obsessive and even counter-productive. Weighing less than once a week makes it too easy to get off track a pound or two at a time.

I also suggest consistency in your weigh-in routine. Weigh yourself at the same time, in the same place, wearing the same amount of clothes. You probably know why; especially if you're like me. I used to use any excuse I could to explain away any added pounds when I weighed in. I was actually pretty good at it. "It's late in the day." "I just ate." "It's that time of the month; you know, water weight." "It's the heavy sweater or blue jeans." "The new watch, that's it! My jewelry . . . the fingernail polish!"

And to be totally honest, to this day I still breathe out before I weigh because I don't want to be responsible for the weight of the air in my lungs! Maybe it's silly, but it's my own routine. Find your own way. With or without the air, weigh weekly...same time, same place, same clothes (or lack thereof).

So many of us have a difficult relationship with the scale. Our pre-weight-loss habit was to avoid it at all costs. We've spent years somehow rationalizing that if we just don't know our weight, it somehow won't be what it really is. But ignorance doesn't change reality. We weigh what we weigh, whether we know the number or not. And knowing the number is a big step toward taking the responsibility that will allow us to control our weight. We must each deter-

TAKE THE
SUCCESS HABITS™ CHALLENGE!

Regular Weighing

1. Select a day and time to weigh yourself each week. Mark it on your day planner and set up an e-reminder message to prompt you.

2. Select a weigh-in location. At home, a doctor's office, hospital or clinic, pharmacy, or gym.

3. Create your manual or online weight-loss chart to track your progress; see Appendix A, Helpful People, Programs, and Products.

Do you know what you weigh? Weigh yourself today.

mine to come to terms with our fear of scales so we can make this habit part of our new lives.

SETTING WEIGHT-LOSS GOALS

So you know exactly what you weigh. Now what? One of the key things I have noticed about the most successful WLS patients is that they always know exactly where they are with their weight at any given time. Prior to surgery, they had a very clear goal in mind. They knew specifically how much they wanted to weigh and how much weight they had to lose to get there. They started with a clear vision of the end in mind. They set a well-defined goal before they began. Faltering patients, on the other hand, seem to simply coast along with no real intent. Not knowing when or if they will ever reach anywhere in particular. Perhaps some of you may remember the tale of Alice In Wonderland and Alice's conversation with the Cheshire Cat.

Alice: "Which way should I go?"

Cat: "That depends on where you are going."

Alice:" I don't know where I am going."

Cat: "Then it doesn't matter which way you go."

- Lewis Carroll, 1872, Through the Looking Glass

To paraphrase, if you don't know where you're going, then any road will take you there. It is so very important that you identify where you are going.

A little later in this chapter I will share with you some ideas and suggestions for setting weight loss goals, but first, I would like to share with you a few stories about the importance of goals in general and share with you some of my personal experiences with goal setting and with goal getting.

Think back to where you were when you were eight years old, back in about second grade. Did you anticipate that your life would look as it now does? Think about what you wanted. What were your dreams? What where your aspirations? When the world was completely open to you, where did you want to go? What did you want to do and be? What did this world of being a grown up look like? I wanted to be married, have a couple of children, and have a house, and a car, and a cat and a dog. And so here I am. Have you, as I have, ever paused and questioned, "Is this it?"

It seems to me that something happens when we grow up: we become very reasonable, very rational, very responsible adults. And we somehow, sometimes, lose the ability to dream those big dreams, to remember those things we wanted when we weren't restricted by the invisible boundaries we now exist within. We start putting limitations on ourselves and we lose that wide-eyed, "anything is possible" kind of mind-set that we had when we were younger.

TOOTSIE

Have you ever been stranded on the side of the road with car problems? It is one of the most infuriating, frustrating, helpless, hopeless, terrible situations, isn't it? I know it is frustrating for anyone to be stranded with car problems, but when your husband is a mechanic, like mine is, there are other things that enter into the equation when something happens to your car. (I had to share that with you so you would know why I could not call my husband when the following situation happened to me.)

It was a beautiful autumn morning. I was up at Snowbird, a ski resort in Utah, speaking at a women's conference. Everything went well again and I was thinking, "Wow, it went great," as I went down to the parking garage and gave my keys to the valet parking guy, who left to get my car. But he didn't come back, and didn't come back and I thought, "Oh man, there was something I was supposed to take care of with my car." But I didn't, and I knew what was wrong with it and I thought, "Ohhh, here we go." Sure enough, the valet parking guy came walking down the ramp, keys in hand.

"Sorry ma'am, your car won't start."

I thought, "Uh oh!" Now... I am a wonderful maiden-in-distress, like the cobbler's children who don't have shoes. Well, the mechanic's wife drives used cars and knows how to do the maiden-in-distress thing. So not only did I have him try again, but I also recruited the bellhop who was just getting off, the night security guy, and also flagged down the maintenance man who had been driving around the parking lot. One at a time these kind men came over, looked a little bit, tinkered a little bit, and said, "Sorry, ma'am, can't help you," and off they'd go. Then I would flag down somebody else. One by one they came. They would try a little bit and one by one they would each say, "You're, like, out of gas, right?"

"No, I am not out of gas;" and so they would give it a good-old college try and say, "Sorry, ma'am, can't help you," and off they'd go.

So, there I stood, all by myself, on this beautiful October Saturday, the sun shining, a little snow glistening, and all by myself with a car that wouldn't go. I knew that all my faith, hope, prayer and positive mental energy was not going to start this car. And so I started to cry. Tears were streaming down my cheeks when out of the corner of my tear-filled eyes I saw an old pickup truck. It was really old, nineteen forty-something, with a square back end, and ply-wood tailgate kind of thing. It had been cleaned up, refurbished and painted shiny, shiny John Deere green. I thought, "You have got to be kidding me." I watched this old truck come around the parking lot and come right in front of me and stop. Then, out of this truck jumped Bob-the-Mechanic and his wife, Tootsie-the-Clown.

Tootsie was in full clown uniform, with very, curly hair, Mickey Mouse ears, long, long eyelashes, a fluffy little skirt and great big feet. She jumped out of the truck and waddled over to me. She didn't say a word. She bent down and with a devastating clown frown, slowly patted her heart as if to show me that her heart was breaking for the terrible, terrible situation that I was in. It's awful to see a clown frown. Without a word, Tootsie got up and climbed back in the truck.

I just stood there in awe when Bob-the-Mechanic asked me a few questions, tinkered with my car a little bit, tweaked it here, tweaked it there and started it! He fired it up, real proud, as he wiped his hands off a little bit. He slammed the hood and came over to me and said, "Well, little lady, we'll just let it idle here for a little bit before we let you go on your way." I thought, "Wow!" He got back in the truck and just then Tootsie-the-Clown jumped back out of the truck again. This time she wore a big clown smile, waddled over, curtsied, bowed as if she were honoring a queen, then handed me a balloon bouquet she had made for me while she waited in the truck. Tootsie smiled, didn't say a word, then climbed back in the truck. I paid them with a bag of pretzels.

Bob-the-Mechanic and Tootsie-the-Clown were delighted and they drove off in the old John Deere green pickup truck, leaving me standing there again, all by myself, tears still streaming, holding my balloon bouquet and flowers; next to my idling car this time. I remember so vividly, looking up to the heavens and exclaiming, "So what's your point?"

I learned a couple of very valuable, unforgettable lessons that day. First, I learned that growing old is a given, but growing up is optional. Bob, wonderful, genuine, good-Samaritan Bob, did something for my car. But Tootsie, that Tootsie, did something for my soul. Tootsie rekindled something in my heart and I started to believe again in clowns, in magic, in laughter, in balloons, and parades, in coloring outside the lines and all those things. I began to think again like I once thought when I was eight or ten. I started to believe in those kinds of things again and I started to believe in myself again. Believing in things like, "Gee, one day maybe I will be a professional public speaker in a size 6." And at 250 pounds it took a pretty big dream, didn't it? A pretty big dream; it seemed like a pretty unrealistic goal.

GOAL SETTING

Let's talk about goal setting for a moment. There are all different kinds of goal-setting packets, journals, logs. Whatever you use, if you are using some method of tracking your dreams and goals, you will surely find some true magic there. Many of you use a day planner or have your goals written in another format. There are all kinds of studies indicating that the most successful people in the world are those who have their goals written down.

Many years ago, I was in a workshop where I participated in a little session on goal setting. It was intended to be a very introspective time. We spent a couple of hours completing the goal setting book, writing down various character traits which we desired, and listing all the things we wanted to learn and do, the places we wanted to go, and all the material things we wanted to have. I followed this assignment very carefully, and as instructed, I listed all of the things I could think of that I wanted. Looking back at that list several years later, I was astonished by what I found; I had obtained everything on my list.

"This is magic!" I thought. The goal-setting gurus are right. If we write goals down, we can accomplish them; I was living proof. A valuable lesson learned, that's for sure, but it was the next realization that has shaped the course of my life since that time. Let me share with you exactly what was on that original wish list. I wanted to have a coat tree for my entryway. I wanted to have new Sunday shoes for my daughter. I wanted to have all of our medical bills paid off, and I wanted to have an Audi 5000. I wrote in parentheses "used okay" (and, yes, that is the car in the Tootsie story).

Looking back I could see that I had obtained everything I had wished for. But then, I wondered, "Wow, this is really something." And then I thought, "Okay, what if I had said I wanted "a new car"? What if I had written down "a bigger

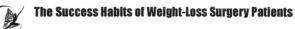

house"? What if I had listed "a pool"? What if "one day I will be a public speaker in a size 6"?

What I learned was a profound truth that has governed my life and my decisions and especially my dreams and goals ever since. The lesson is this:

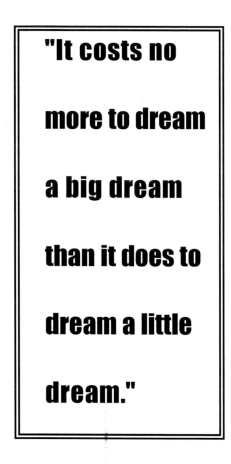

"It costs no more to dream a big dream than it does to dream a little dream."

May I challenge you to take the time to list your wildest dreams, all of the things that you have forgotten about. As you do keep this story in mind:

When my son was eight years old, in second grade, he was given a writing assignment. The assignment was to finish this sentence: "If I were in charge of the world . . . " This is what he said:

"If I were in charge of the world I would cancel school,

drugs, and cocaine. If I were in charge of the world there would be no homework or fried chicken, and if I were in charge of the world a person who forgot to comb his hair and forgot to go to the bathroom before class would still be allowed to be in charge of the world." Quite interesting, don't you think?

You see, you are in charge of your world. As you write down some of the things you want out of life, keep your mind open to the many possibilities; simply refuse to limit yourself.

Remember when Mary Poppins jumped into the pavement picture? What would your world look like if you could have it just the way you want it? Write down some of those things. Next, write down as many details as possible and visualize your goal as a reality, in complete detail. Be specific.

Before you begin to set your goals, I encourage you to do this little activity. Picture yourself in the future; ten years in the future.

What does your life look like? Where do you live? What do you do each day? How old are you ten years from now? How old are your children in ten years? And here's a scary thought: How old is your spouse or partner going to be ten years from now?

Once you have a clear picture of that future in mind, ask

yourself these questions: Are you headed in the right direction? Are you on your way where you want to be and will your life look like you think it should in ten years?

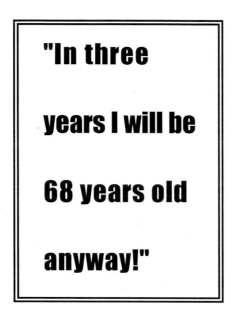

"In three

years I will be

68 years old

anyway!"

To get where you want to be, where do you need to be in five years? Yes, that's right; half way there. What does that look like? Now, if you intend to be "there" in five years, what do you need to do to move you closer to your lifetime goals THIS year? This month? Today?

Stress comes into our lives when we spend our time, our money and our energy doing things that are NOT getting us closer to our goals. We spend so much time simply existing, dealing with whatever life throws at us. Instead of simply responding to the circumstances of your life, may I encourage you to do some planning. Identify those things in life that you truly want. And then take steps every single day in the right, well-defined direction toward your goals.

Hyrum Smith, president and founder of The Franklin Covey Company, relates a story about overhearing a conversation his mother had with one of her girlfriends. She was 65 years old at the time and was telling her friend, "I am going to go back to the University of Hawaii and get another degree." Her friend exclaimed, "What do you mean, Another degree? It will take you three years to get another degree. You are 65 years old. In three years you will be 68 years old!" Hyrum's mother calmly and wisely replied, "In three years I will be 68 years old anyway!"

> "If you limit your choices to only that which seems possible or reasonable then you disconnect yourself from what you truly want and all that is left is a compromise."
> — Robert Fritz

The time between now and ten years from now will go by, one way or the other. You can either be closer to your goals or further away from them, but, make no mistake about it, the time will go by.

Let me share with you one of my favorite stories about a man by the name of Larry Walters.

Larry Walters was a thirty-three year old truck driver, who wanted to fly. He had big, huge dreams of being able to fly. For as long as he could remember, he wanted to fly; to be able to just rise right up in the air and see for a long way. The time, money, education and opportunity to be a pilot weren't his. Hang gliding was too dangerous and any good place for gliding was too far away. So he spent many of his Saturday and Sunday afternoons sitting in his backyard, in his old aluminum lawn chair; sitting there, drinking his six pack of beer, looking up at the birds, wishing he could fly.

The next time we hear about Larry Walters, he's in the news because he was flying, at last. And he's still sitting in his old aluminum lawn chair, to which he had tied forty-five helium-filled weather surplus balloons. He had a parachute, a CB radio, two peanut butter and jelly sandwiches, a pack of beer, and a BB gun to shoot the balloons so he could come back down. (Can you imagine his wife saying, "You're going to what?!") Now the reason the media was involved is that Larry was not just hovering over his neighborhood in his backyard. He had shot up eleven thousand feet, right into the approach corridor to the Los Angeles International Airport. A pilot saw him and said, "I don't know what this is, but you need to get it out of my way." But there was Larry Walters, flying at last. Now, as the story goes, he shot enough balloons so that he landed safely in a field somewhere. The media interrogated him after landing, asking, "Why did you do this?" And Larry said, "Well, you can't just sit there."

And they asked, "Oh, were you scared?" And he said, "Wonderfully so." And the third reporter asked him, "Well, Larry, are you going to do this again?" And he said, "Nope."

What a huge dream ... A huge dream!

Another example of dreaming big dreams and setting unrealistic goals is Grandma Moses. Were you aware that she did not even start to paint until she was 84 years old?

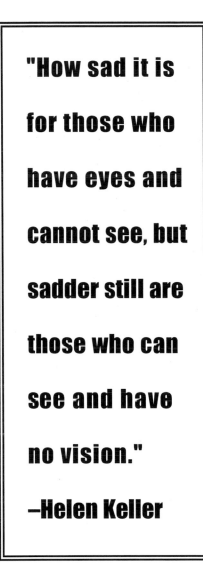

"How sad it is for those who have eyes and cannot see, but sadder still are those who can see and have no vision."

–Helen Keller

I encourage you to dream big dreams, huge dreams, unbelievable dreams and remember that it will cost you no more to dream a big dream than it will to dream a little dream?

Helen Keller said this:"How sad it is for those who have eyes and cannot see, but sadder still are those who can see and have no vision."

You alone are responsible for what your future looks like; You alone are responsible for creating your life's vision. As you do, always remember these words from the movie, Thelma and Louise, "You get what you settle for." Learn to settle for nothing but the very best for yourself. For additional information on setting goals, you may enjoy BSCI's Goal Getting Book.

WEIGHT LOSS GOALS

There is a folk tale about a traveler roaming the countryside. He stopped at an intersection and asked a local farmer, "How long will it take me to get to the next town?" "I don't know," replied the farmer, "that depends on how fast you walk!"

Many prospective and new patients ask, "When will I reach my goal weight?" Well, that depends on how fast you lose. Predicting an exact weight-loss goal date is nearly an impossible task. Everyone is different. "How much should I weigh?" and "How much can I lose?" are also questions that are frequently asked, and they are questions that are difficult for someone else to determine. Keeping in mind that the average weight loss after weight-loss surgery is 100 to 120 pounds in the first year, we have observed the following:

- The more weight you have to lose the longer it will take.

- Men lose weight faster than women.

- The optimum time for weight loss is during the first 12 to 18 months after surgery.

- Weight loss will be rapid at first and then slow down.

- Some people lose steadily, while others have periods of rapid weight-loss alternating with plateaus.

When you begin this weight-loss journey, may I encourage you to set two goals: first, a goal weight; and second, a warning weight of 5 to 7 pounds above your goal.

Do you have both of those numbers in mind? If not, here are a few suggestions: To set a goal weight, begin by asking these questions:

- Have I ever felt good about my weight? If so, what did I weigh at that time?

- What is the suggested healthy weight range for someone like me, as listed in the Metropolitan Life Tables or Body Mass Index charts? (See Appx B.)

- What weight range do I think I would feel comfortable with?

- What size do I think is right for my body type and height?

- Do I know someone of similar frame and height that weighs what I want to weigh?

Now, set a total weight-loss goal and a one-year weight-loss goal. Keep in mind that you are likely to have a few pounds of additional loose skin after you lose a significant amount of weight and you may also have a higher bone density than a "normal" person, due to the excess weight you've been carrying around. Both of these factors can result in needless disappointment if you set an unreasonably low weight-loss goal or a goal date that is too ambitious.

Joe, a new patient fresh out of surgery, is a good example of a guy with unreasonable expectations. Joe attended support group meeting on the night we introduced our weight-loss progress chart to the group. (See Appendix C.)

We printed charts for anyone in attendance who wanted one. Those who wanted a chart were asked to fill out a simple form indicating their start weight, start date, goal weight, and goal date.

Using these four data points we created a chart for each patient, showing what their average weight-loss progress should be at any time between their start date and their goal date. The chart provides an excellent visual indication for patients who live by the Success Habits™ principles that their weight-loss progress is on track. It helps reduce needless worry when a patient encounters a plateau if they can see they are well ahead of their projected weight-loss at that point. Having the opportunity to see the charts of other people who have gone before them also makes it easier to see their weight-loss pattern as being typical when they encounter a plateau.

Joe turned in his form, indicating that he intended to lose 300 pounds in one year! Joe weighed 460 pounds and was planning to weigh 160 pounds (the same amount he weighed in high school) 12 months later. We made two charts for Joe: one as he requested, and one showing his 300-pound weight loss occurring over two years; a more reasonable time period.

You should keep track of your individual weight-loss in whatever format you feel most comfortable with. Just be sure to evaluate your progress regularly and plan to set intermediate goals as needed.

TAKE THE
SUCCESS HABITS™ CHALLENGE!

Setting Weight-loss Goals

1. Gather any records you can of your weight through the years; old Weight Watcher® logs, doctor's charts, health records, etc. Review and analyze your ups and downs and see if you can identify what your circumstances were when: You were at your lowest, highest, healthiest, etc.

2. To help you select a goal weight, try to select a particular size that you would like to be. Find someone of your same height and or build who is about the size you would like to be and estimate their weight.

You may appreciate some of the charts, progress records and journals listed at the back of this book in our section titled "Helpful Products, People and Programs."

Connie's Story - Gastric Bypass

I was not always overweight. I was very active throughout my childhood and teen years. In high school I was the captain of the swim team and in great shape. I stayed fit until my junior year of college when genetics, combined with poor eating habits, began to catch up to me. The changes that occurred not only affected my physical appearance but also my self-confidence. I've always had a great deal of self confidence; however, with the added weight, I was more cautious of my actions. I never wanted to be perceived as a "big, pushy woman."

By the time I was 23 years old, I was conservative about my interactions with people and self-conscious when participating in activities that I had previously enjoyed. I felt that I was too fat to ride a bike, even though the exercise would have been good for me. I would no longer go out dancing with my friends because I didn't want to be the center of attention (in a bad way). There were two activities that I continued to participate in; golfing and swimming. Eventually I even gave up swimming.

As I got older I felt worse. My physical health was compromised and my mental health was bruised. I fell into the

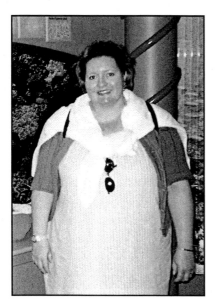

all-too-familiar cycle of
dieting, not seeing
results, and then com-
forting myself with
food. This pattern con-
tinued until 1999 when I
was 34 years old. It was
a pivotal year for me
because I was forced to
look at my future
through the life and
death of my father.

There is a significant
history of heart disease
in my father's family. My grandfather had his first heart
attack at the age of 41; he died of a heart attack at the age
of 67. My father had his first echocardiogram at the age of
44; he died of a heart attack at 57.

My grandfather was the type of man who did what the
doctor told him to do. After his first heart attack, he quit
smoking and watched his weight. My father was a different
type of patient; he did not do what his doctor told him to do.
My father had type two diabetes, high cholesterol and was
obese. He was in constant conflict and denial over the
severity of his health problems. Before my father passed
away, he was on life support. His cardiologist talked sin-

cerely and seriously to me about making an appointment and having my heart and health evaluated.

I had a treadmill test and it was determined that my heart was in good shape considering my weight and the family predisposition to heart disease; however, I had high cholesterol. The doctor gave me a diet to follow for two weeks. I followed the diet down to the smallest detail. After two weeks I returned to the doctor's office to find that my cholesterol had not improved at all. The doctor encouraged me to give the diet two more weeks. Again, there was no improvement.

The next step was cholesterol-lowering medication. I was only 34. I did not want to start taking prescriptions to control my cholesterol. I had been thinking about weight-loss surgery and I asked the cardiologist what his opinion of the procedure was. He warned me of the risks involved but also noted that at my current pace I wouldn't live a long life.

I talked to my husband about the procedure. He was very supportive and understanding. My husband has relatives that had the procedure with successful results and my husband's overall response was, "If you die of a heart attack like your father did, I will have a hard time dealing with it if you didn't do everything you could have done to avoid having a heart attack." At that moment I knew that I needed to do more research on my own to determine if weight-loss surgery would be the best solution for me.

It never fails to amaze me; as soon as weight-loss surgery is mentioned there are two polarizing opinions. One side knows someone who had a horrible experience: a long and unpleasant recovery, and the person ended up gaining all of the weight back or worse, the person died. The other side knows someone who was very successful with a new approach to food and overall health improvements.

While I was researching I would listen to these opinions. If I heard a story with unpleasant results, I would ask for the name of the unfortunate victim of this heinous procedure. In two out of three situations, these were people whom I knew personally, people I considered friends. I approached these people honestly about my intentions. I wanted to know why they felt this procedure had failed them or why they had failed to be successful.

Overwhelmingly the response was, "It wasn't a cure-all or a quick fix." These friends were candid and open with their responses to my questions. I appreciated their answers and humility when I faced them with unpleasant questions.

In order for my research to be balanced, I asked for the names of people considered successful. This time the response was different, "It was a complete lifestyle change." The stories that I heard were uplifting and inspiring. The responses were every bit as honest. I heard about getting sick from eating the wrong foods too soon after surgery and other common problems that weight-loss surgery patients face.

After I finished my personal research, I began to do professional research. This step was easy; I had been told about the amazing results that Dr. Sherman Smith and the other surgeons in his practice were having. It was time for me to schedule my first appointment with Dr. Smith. I was determined to be successful. I had all the facts I needed and I knew I could change my life.

Because of the controversial nature of the weight-loss surgery procedure, I was reluctant to tell anyone that I was going to have surgery. I told only my immediate family with the threat of severe consequences if anyone mentioned that I was going to have surgery. The reason for this was because my mind was made up. I didn't want to hear any negative opinions or arguments about my decision. The same was true of my coworkers. I only confided in my bosses because I needed to schedule time off from work.

I had surgery in June 2000. It couldn't have come sooner. I was constantly out of breath, I felt horrible about myself, and I was wearing a tight size 28. I was at my all-time highest weight, 305 pounds, one month before surgery. Once my surgery was scheduled, I wouldn't get on a scale again until after I was released from the hospital. It's very possible that I weighed more than 305 by the time I had surgery, but I'll never know for sure.

I must admit I was very fortunate. I didn't have complications and my pain was minimal. Of course I had the same fear that all patients have the first time the nurse announces,

"You must go to the bathroom on your own." Once I got out of bed, went to the bathroom and then got back into bed, I knew I was going to be okay. Then, I gave my permission for family and friends to tell others.

Since my surgery I have been open and honest about how wonderful the procedure has worked for me and how lucky I am to have had it. Not long after my surgery I became a Bariatric Support Center volunteer at St. Mark's Hospital. I've met many amazing patients and I'm always inspired by their commitment to change their lives. The patients I visit keep me focused on my future by reminding me where I once was.

I have a new lease on life and am grateful to Dr. Sherman Smith for the tool he has given me. I also know I must use the tool wisely. My accountability is foremost in my thoughts and actions; I know if I am unsuccessful, it is because of my actions and behavior.

I continue to have the same struggles I had before surgery. If I have a stressful moment, I look for food to calm my nerves and lend comfort. However, I'm smarter now. I only keep acceptable snacks in my office and I think about how much time has passed since my last glass of water. By the time I wait 30 minutes to eat my stress snack, I'm no longer stressed and I'm able to avoid unnecessary snacking.

It's been over two years since my surgery, and my health has improved tremendously. My cholesterol levels are normal, I'm never out of breath and I'm in great shape (again). I've taken salsa-dancing classes and I started running 5K races. I don't like to run, but I love the feeling of accomplishment I have when I finish a race.

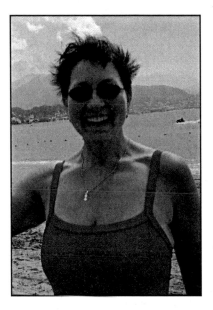

And now I'm a much better golfer. I'm even the person in the group who grumbles when my friends want to rent golf carts. I enjoy hearing encouraging and uplifting compliments from my friends and family. And most of all I love it when I hear, "You are so thin."

TAKE THE
SUCCESS HABITS™ CHALLENGE!

Personal Accountability

1. Get a new do for the new you! Treat yourself to a new hair cut or color. Enjoy all of the complements and just smile when people say, "Something is different about you!"

2. Find a great new outfit on a budget! Take your nice clothes to a consignment shop or sell them online at our Clothing Exchange Forum (see Appendix A, Helpful People, Programs, and Products). Use the proceeds to buy something new for you now and something new for you to wear later, when you are a few sizes smaller!

3. The best way to lighten up and to improve your attitude is to help someone else. Share a story or an uplifting thought with another patient or supporter. Post your story or thought online and share your success with others.

Maral's Story - LapBand® - Toronto, Canada

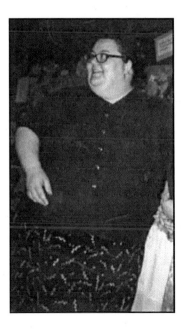

It began three years ago with hopes, dreams, and a passionate desire for change. A desire that was greater than the fear of it. Continuing to stay where I was with all my disabilities was the greatest fear of all. There was a definite consciousness that I could no longer continue the way I was….and I made the decision to have Laparoscopic Band Surgery.

It was a one baby step at a time. I remember that it took great courage for me to stand on the scale for my pre-operative assessment - 427 pounds. I had to allow myself to first, feel overwhelmed, then accept it, then stay with myself and choose to continue to take the necessary steps to better health.

The learning curve continued to develop over days, weeks, months and eventually years…Learning to accept my tool and working with it was bitter sweet. Sweet, because I could finally taste life for what it was and experience it, not just as an outside observer, but as an active participant. I began to feel comfortable giving into a hugs without the fear of being too heavy for the other person. I began to enjoy conversations with acquaintances and finally felt like what I had to say was worthwhile. I became more confident with myself and comfortable with all the changes I was making. As more weight cam off, I experienced mobility once again, being able to move my arms and legs and embark on many adventures without physical limitations.

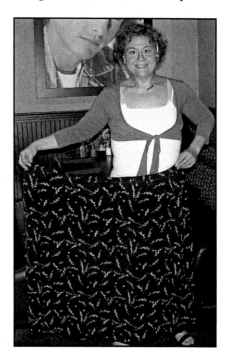

Bitter, because with the peeling of my layers, came the realization that appetites are much more than physiological needs. I felt joy in feeling satiety, fullness, restriction. I felt sadness in knowing that I had emotional and spiritual needs that needed tending. I realized that I could no longer neglect parts of me that needed to be acknowledged and nurtured. I allowed myself to experience all my sensations through guided imagery, meditations, journal reflections, group support, yoga and cardio activities

Today, I have lost 280 pounds with the Laparoscopic Band. This success has allowed me to be able to make choices again. I am making commitments to myself and enjoying inner peace and love. I am building relationships. I am accepting obstacles and challenges as all part of the process. I am showing myself time and time again that I can do it. I am discovering strengths and setting the foundation for further successes.

I hold gratitude in my heart of hearts for all that I am and all that I will become.

Success Habits™ Principle 1
Personal Accountability

DAILY CHECK-UP QUESTIONS

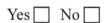

I took responsibility for my actions
today.   Yes ☐ No ☐

I feel in control of myself today.   Yes ☐ No ☐

I will do my best to master the
Success Habits™ principles
one more day.   Yes ☐ No ☐

Portion Control

"I understand the importance of satiety
and listen to my body's signals."

From a personal standpoint, one of the key elements contributing to my success with weight-loss surgery is that my body feels full and satisfied when I have eaten very little food. I recall prior to surgery coming up with several solutions for my weight problems. After countless fad diets and "wonder" drugs, I decided to be hypnotized. Yes! That's what I would do; I would have them hypnotize me and tell me I only had a two-ounce stomach! (Well, I decided not to go through with that.) Next, I decided I would just cut back and reduce my portion size. That was it! I would just eat like a weight-loss surgery patient and the results would be the same, right?

With all the discipline I could muster, I spent several months eating smaller portions and did lose a bit of weight, but as you know, when you have 125 pounds to lose, a few months of concentrated effort is just not enough. So, why didn't that work? It seems like it should have. Such a simple principle: just eat less! Why wasn't it working? And then it hit me. As an experienced dieter, I knew that even if I was disciplined enough to reduce my portions and eat less than 800 calories each day, my body would go into starvation mode and respond by storing everything; even the lettuce, it seemed. Through the years I have counseled with many people investigating weight-loss surgery. We often talk about all of the diets, pills, powders, exercise programs and behavior modification programs, both the reasonable and the far-fetched. Often I've found that attempts at "portion control" are common. And the results? well, they were the same as mine. Perhaps you, too, have tried to just cut down, eating small amounts which left you feeling unsatisfied and frustrated, especially when little or no weight loss was the result. The key difference in my success with portion control efforts now, as compared to my futile efforts prior to surgery, is that now after eating a small amount my body feels full. As satiety sets in, I feel well and comfortably satisfied and that all-important signal is sent to my brain telling it that I am full and my body metabolizes food like it should. Since weight-loss surgery I have found time and time again, that if I will just listen to my body, it will help me know what to eat, when to eat and how much to eat.

In this chapter we'll learn a little about how our digestive tract works, discuss satiety and its importance in our weight loss and maintenance, and study some tips to avoid grazing and learn how to establish good eating habits.

STOMACH SIZE CHANGES

The sensors that send the signal of satiety to the brain are located in the upper curvature of the stomach. An obese person's stomach has the capacity to hold 1 1/2 to 2, and sometimes, as much as 3 quarts of food at one time. With that in mind it's easy to see how an obese person is able to eat and drink so much before feeling full. One of the primary benefits of having weight-loss surgery is the new physical ability to feel full and satisfied on very little food, thereby helping to reduce the amount of calories we consume.

Bariatric surgical procedures are, of course, designed to create a new small stomach pouch that limits the amount of food that can be consumed at each sitting.

Throughout the first several months following surgery, as this small, newly-created stomach pouch heals, it expands a bit and the scarring around the anastamosis (pouch outlet) relaxes and stretches. Within a year's time, a two-ounce pouch can accommodate more volume. Thereafter, it will usually hold approximately six to eight ounces (3/4 cup-one cup) of food at a time.

It is important to learn to listen to your body and to recognize what "full" feels like. It's vital to learn to stop eating when your pouch is full and it is equally important to learn to eat enough. This is a common challenge for new patients.

There have been some differences through the years regarding the exact size of the stomach pouch. In earlier years (Late 1970's), the pouch size was approximately three or four ounces (89-119 ml). Now 2 ounces (32 ml) is com-

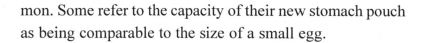

mon. Some refer to the capacity of their new stomach pouch as being comparable to the size of a small egg.

Others, like Dr. Robert Marema of Ft. Lauderdale, Florida, a patient himself, teaches his patients that the size of their thumb is the size of their new pouch. Do you know what size your stomach is? Do you know how much it can hold? Do you know how much it should hold? These are important things for you to know.

Knowing and understanding the importance of properly sized meal portions during both the weight-loss phase and the weight management phase is a key factor to your success. Successful patients know that, in addition to making sure they don't overeat, they must also make sure they eat enough to feel comfortably satisfied.

Eating until we feel full at meals ensures that we get that very important feeling of satiety. Without it, we feel hungry and pretty soon we are constantly snacking or grazing throughout the day. Grazing throughout the day results in a higher calorie intake for the day than we would have eaten if we had focused on eating three high quality meals, where we ate until we were full.

SATIETY

It's important for us to begin by learning what satiety is and how it is achieved. To do so, we must first understand the differences between hunger and appetite.

TAKE THE
SUCCESS HABITS™ CHALLENGE!

Stomach Size Changes

1. Take the Cottage Cheese Test to determine the size of your stomach pouch. (See page 66.)

2. Measure the amount of food you can eat at breakfast, lunch and dinner and record your results.

3. Notice the volume that "normal" people can eat and drink at one time. Estimate that in cups or ounces.

HUNGER is the primary physiological drive to find food to eat. It is driven by several internal and external forces that work together to provide the body with food in order to extinguish the desire to eat. Hunger is the true need for nourishment.

APPETITE, however, is simply the desire to eat and has little to do with nourishment. Most weight-loss surgeries are restrictive procedures that allow the patient to have the feeling of satiety; to feel full and satisfied on very little food.

SATIETY is the state of being full or gratified to or beyond the point of satisfaction. (To learn more about Hunger and Satiety, you may enjoy BSCI's Maintenance Mentality Book, by Janean Hall).

The feeling of satisfaction or fullness is only one of the factors influencing the level of our satiety. There are both internal and learned factors which influence how often we have the desire to eat.

1. Internal Cues

Eating to survive - real hunger
Cravings for sweets
Inherent set point - genetics

2. Learned Eating Cues

> Social or ritual eating
> Habitual eating
> Food - mood

Additionally, the foods we choose to eat play an important part in how long we are able to stay full. Dr. Susanne Holt, researcher, conducted a study at the University of Sidney to establish a ranking system for different foods based on their ability to satisfy. Her findings included the following interesting information.

- Beans and lentils contain anti-nutrients, which delay their absorption so they make people feel full longer.

- Fatty foods are not satisfying even though people expect them to be.

- The more protein a food contains, the longer it will satisfy.

(Reference: Apex Fitness Group)

Several years ago I had the privilege of hearing bariatric surgeon, Dr. Laytham Flanagan speak at the ASBS (American Society for Bariatric Surgery) Conference. His speech was titled "Understanding the Function of the Small Gastric Pouch."

Generally, the ASBS Plenary Session presentations are intense, detailed discussions about surgical technique or rare cases and they are usually outside my area of interest. But when Doctor Flanagan began his presentation, I tuned right in. As I listened intently, I found myself nodding my head and thinking, "He gets it!" He was verbalizing some of the same thoughts that I had as a patient. He seemed to understand, and was presenting research to back up his belief, that long-term success was linked directly to the patient's ability to effectively use the stomach pouch to stay full and satisfied for as long as possible. With Dr. Flanagan's permission, I have enclosed excerpts from his research here:

(Excerpts from "Understanding the Function of the Small Gastric Pouch." By Latham Flanagan, Jr., M.D., F.A.C.S.)

From our earliest experiences in bariatric surgery, we have been intrigued with the question, "How does our operation cause weight loss and maintenance?" As we talked to the public, and even our medical peers, it became evident that a common concept of the uninformed is that the small gastric pouch simply mechanically restricts intake, preventing the post-op patient from eating too much. Indeed, superficially, it may appear that way, especially in the first 3 to 9 months after surgery. Yet, a short experience with following our patients shows us that with a meal size of even 3 to 5 ounces, certain patients will stop losing weight and start to regain. We also note that 2 to 5 or more years after surgery, certain patients seem to have a large meal volume (6 to 10 ounces) but still maintain good weight control without an obnoxious degree of hunger. It has become clear with experience that the essential principle of weight control is the achievement of satiety, or the absence of abnormal hunger, associated with the ingestion of the appropriate number of calories sufficient to meet the person's need.

If adequate satiety is achieved, our patients are successful; they fail if that satiety is not achieved. When patients "fail" there is a tendency, even among bariatric surgeons, to pass it off as "noncompliance." Certainly, this can be an appropriate evaluation in a few persons who are not willing to accept responsibility for the lifestyle changes necessary to make the small gastric pouch function properly.

But, is this the problem for the majority? I think not. When failure does occur, it is usually the inability to maintain the post meal satiety long enough to prevent snacking before the next meal time arrives.

THREE PRINCIPLES FOR GAINING AND MAINTAINING SATIETY

1. The pouch needs to be truly filled with adequate wall distention with each meal (i.e. no snacking).

2. Keep the pouch filled over time and slow down the emptying time (by eating solid foods and avoiding liquids for fifteen minutes before and one and one half to two hours after eating.) We understand this to be the most important lifestyle change after the weight-loss surgery procedure.

3. Finally, adequate protein is needed with each meal. We emphasize the need for three meals a day including breakfast (defined as the first meal of the day which is eaten within one to two hours after arising). The "enemies" are high calorie liquids. Snacking and consuming high calorie liquids cheat the patient because the calories are taken in without offering significant satiety.

The following are observations that may have an effect on the function of the weight-loss surgery pouch:

We have come to understand that the accomplishment of satiety, or suppression of hunger, is fundamental to the success or failure of bariatric operations.

We have come to understand that success relates anatomically to creating a small pouch that remains relatively small and a small outlet that remains relatively small.

Meal volumes much larger than ten to twelve ounces usually result in failure of weight maintenance.

The use of the thick, less distensible lesser curve of the stomach is believed to be important by many surgeons.

Satiety is achieved by increasing the tension on the gastric pouch wall, thus stimulating the stretch receptors.

Maintaining satiety is dependent upon maintaining some portion of that stretch for an undefined period of time.

For either the weight-loss surgery or the banded gastroplasty, almost all patients have a profound satiety 24 hours a day in the first six months or so after their bariatric surgical procedure. They do not redevelop a normal appetite preceding the next meal until six to twelve months postoperatively.

If for any reason the patient is NPO ["nothing by mouth"] for a significant period of time (eight to twelve hours), profound hunger will be experienced.

In the mature pouch (one or more years post-op), the satiety period correlates with the amount of solid food the patient eats (i.e. a patient eating a greater amount of solid foods will experience a longer period of satiety).

Almost all patients after the weight-loss surgery procedure, and most patients after the vertical banded gastroplasty, achieve fifteen to twenty-five minutes of satiety after simply rapidly drinking water to a point of fullness, or "water loading."

Some patients fail the banded gastroplasties in association with shifting their diets to mostly liquids or soft solids, the "soft calorie syndrome," which can cause hunger before the next scheduled meal. This often results in snacking between meals with weight gain as the consequence.

Responsible patients who carefully follow the guidelines and principles for using their "pouch/tool" continue to have reliable and progressive weight-loss and weight-maintenance.

Patients who approach or become underweight one to two years following bariatric surgery can reverse their weight loss by reversing the principles of using their pouch.

–Latham Flanagan, Jr., M.D.

May I reiterate what I believe to be the key point of Dr. Flanagan's article? "We have come to understand that the accomplishment of satiety, or suppression of hunger, is fundamental to the success or failure of bariatric operations."

So how do you measure up? Are you accomplishing the feeling of satiety at each meal? Do you know how big your stomach pouch is? Would you like to know? Nearly every patient I have worked with through the years has been curious to know just exactly how big their stomach pouch is.

The following technique is used by bariatric surgeons and patients to determine the functional size of a patient's stomach pouch.

The idea for this technique began with Dr. E. E. Mason, who suggested at one of the Iowa Bariatric symposia in the early 1980s. He suggested that it might be useful to ask patients to eat cottage cheese in a structured manner to attempt to determine their functional meal volume at different times after their surgery. Dr. Flanagan is known for his research and experience in implementing the "Cottage Cheese Test." This test is designed to be a standardized measurement of the physical size of the stomach pouch of a weight-loss surgery patient.

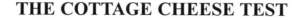

THE COTTAGE CHEESE TEST

STEP 1: *Purchase a container of small curd, low-fat cottage cheese.*

STEP 2: *Begin the test with a full container of cottage cheese, and perform the test in the morning before eating anything else. This will be your breakfast on that day.*

STEP 3: *Eat fairly quickly until you feel full (less than five minutes). Note that the small soft curds do not require much chewing. You are eating rapidly so you will fill the pouch before there is time for any food to flow out of it.*

STEP 4: *After eating your "fill" of cottage cheese, you will be left with a partially eaten container that has empty space where cottage cheese used to be.*

STEP 5: *Measure the volume of cottage cheese you have eaten by filling a two cup (16 fl. oz.) measuring cup with water. Pour water into the container of cottage cheese until the water level rises to the original top level of the cottage cheese.*

RESULTS: *The amount of water poured into the container is the functional size of your pouch.*

Dr. Flanagan's research indicates that the average volume of the mature stomach pouch of a Roux-en-Y patient measured by this method is 5.5 ounces (163 ml).

TAKE THE
SUCCESS HABITS™ CHALLENGE!

Hunger and Satiety

1. Begin a weight-loss journal. Start by writing down those times when you think you are hungry and the circumstances surrounding those times. Have you eaten recently? Are you craving something in particular? Analyze your findings.

2. Make a list of those foods that cause you to feel full. Which foods stay with you the longest? Then make a list of the foods that don't seem to fill you up or stay with you long. Adjust your meal plans accordingly.

3. Slow down! It takes time for your mind to recognize the signal of satiety. Time yourself to be sure you are taking 20 to 30 minutes to eat each meal.

Additionally, he reached the conclusion that "sizes ranging up to 9 ounces have NO IMPACT on the person's success in weight-loss."

This means that unless your pouch holds a volume greater than 9 ounces (267 ml), the exact size of your pouch is not a critical factor in whether or not you can lose your excess weight and then manage your weight as time progresses.

ADOPTING GOOD EATING HABITS

The stomach's ability to aid in the digestive process is greatly limited following weight-loss surgery. It's important for us to understand just how our new stomach functions and also understand how we must change our eating habits in order to maximize the effectiveness of our digestive process.

Prior to Weight-loss Surgery: The stomach, located in the upper abdomen just below the diaphragm, is a sac-like structure with strong, muscular walls. The main function of the stomach is to process and transport food. To aid in digestion, the stomach (a muscle) contracts about three times per minute, churning the food and mixing it with gastric juice, thus aiding in the digestive process.

After Weight-loss Surgery: Following weight-loss surgery, the newly created stomach pouch has limited capacity to assist with digestion. It does not contract and expand and no longer churns and mixes as it once did. Consequently, it is essential that patients learn how to eat properly in order to aid in digestion, avoid discomfort, and maximize absorption.

Here are a few tips that patients have found to be helpful in establishing good eating habits:

• **Eat only** This takes discipline, but it is an important habit to incorporate. Learn to sit down and simply eat and enjoy your meals. Don't eat on the run or while doing anything else.

• **Eat slowly** To avoid discomfort and aid in eating proper quantities, it is important to take at least 20 to 30 minutes to eat each meal.

• **Chew food thoroughly** Make a conscious effort to chew your food thoroughly to aid in the digestive process.

• **Don't drink while you are eating** It's important to avoid drinking with your meals in order to ensure that you are eating the proper quantities of good, solid food. More on eating and drinking together will be discussed in the next chapter, "Proper Drinking."

• **Use a small plate and small utensils** Our eyes are often bigger than our stomachs (especially now!). Using

TAKE THE
SUCCESS HABITS™ CHALLENGE!

Developing Good Eating Habits

1. Take inventory of your eating habits. List three things that you feel are good habits and three things that are poor habits. Select one to work on.

2. Know for sure how long it takes you to eat a meal. Time yourself at breakfast, lunch, and dinner. How does your time measure up to your target of 20 to 30 minutes?

a small plate and small utensils will help you keep portion sizes down and you'll waste less food.

• **Measure** Two to four ounces of food is a good rule of
thumb for new patients. The volume you can eat will
increase during the first year, until you can eat about six
to eight ounces at one year and thereafter. It's easy to
lose track of just how much you are eating and so it's a
good idea to keep things in check by measuring periodically.

• **Eat protein first** In the chapter on nutrition we go into
detail about the importance of protein, but for now,
always eating protein first ensures good nutrition and
helps to curb the appetite for other filling, but less nutri-
tious, foods.

THE DANGERS OF GRAZING

We are encouraged to plan our meals in advance; to
shop for the things we need to ensure that we have high
quality, well-balanced meals. We should eat three meals
each day and avoid eating between meals. But is this how
we're really eating?

Grazing is a common behavior in people who regain
weight following weight-loss surgery. "Grazing" is a term
commonly used to describe mindless or unplanned eating,
reminiscent of cattle in a pasture continually eating grass

throughout the day.

Many faltering patients report eating haphazardly off and on throughout the day, instead of eating deliberate, well thought-out meals. They eat a little here and a little there and, consequently, never feel truly hungry and never feel completely full. This becomes a problem because, as we discussed earlier, feeling full is essential to our well-being and has a direct correlation to our long-term weight control success.

While weight-loss surgery patients cannot physically eat too much at one time, it is possible to eat the wrong foods all day long, and that can result in consuming more than is needed in a given day. Remember the weight control ratio: Calories-In vs. Calories-Out. If we eat more than is expended in energy, we gain weight. By grazing, little by little, snack by snack, bite by bite, unwanted pounds will easily sneak up on us. The consequence of nibbling is extra weight.

But understanding why we should eat regular meals and keep from grazing is only half of the battle. There are many factors that can make the ideal difficult to achieve. The hurried lifestyle most of us are living makes it harder to plan and prepare well thought-out meals. It is not often easy to take the time to sit down, relax and enjoy a peaceful meal. We know what we should and shouldn't do; we know the dangers; so how do we break the habit of grazing? Here are some questions for you to consider and some tips to ponder, from patients who have learned to successfully avoid grazing and have, instead, adopted good eating habits.

What time of day am I most likely to graze?

It's likely that the temptation to graze comes at the same time each day. By identifying when these tempting times are, you can anticipate them and redirect your activities as needed to arrange for different circumstances, surroundings, etc.

What activities might be encouraging me to graze?

When the temptation to graze hits, observe what is going on around you. Are you watching TV? At the movies? Driving in your car? Identify these "at-risk" times and make changes or prepare for them in advance by removing poor foods and having better food choices available.

What am I eating at these times and how did I get it?

Are you eating a particular food simply because it's there? If certain foods are difficult for you to pass up, don't buy them! And don't allow others to bring them into the house. Making this decision once at the grocery store will prevent you from having to decide again every time you walk by the kitchen. It's also important to prepare for times when you need a little pick-me-up. Plan for them in advance by having snacks available that are good for you, such as cheese sticks, jerky, vegetables, nuts, etc.

What type of food am I craving (i.e. salty, sweet, chewy, cold, crunchy)?

Learning to listen to your body is one of the most important skills you can develop for a healthy lifestyle. Knowing what your body is craving may give you clues about what your body needs. Perhaps you know the feeling of wanting something salty, or sweet. Pay close attention and try to identify just what it is that your body is telling you. (You may find that it is not hunger, but rather thirst.)

How am I feeling when I'm tempted to graze?

Often our cravings are to satisfy emotional needs. Notice how you feel when you are wanting to snack. Are you tired? Stressed? Bored? Anxious or nervous? Be aware of these emotions, then identify and practice alternative ways to soothe them.

Cara's Story - Vertical Sleeve Gastrectomy

It says its right there in my baby book under First Words. Like most babies who utter "ma-ma" and "da-da". I managed to have one of my first words to be "COOKIE". I always loved food and I probably always will. I was a chubby kid starting around age 7 and although very active in dance I remained chubby. As a young girl growing up in

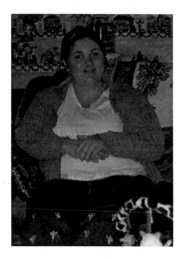

the 80's I became victim to the diet fads. From Nutrisystem® to drops you put under your tongue. By age 13 I was an expert. I was on my first one at age 11. I can remember the ridicule at the breakfast table as my mother (bless her heart because I know it was out of love) measured my cereal with a scale and a scoop, while my skinny brat brother gorged himself across from me. At snack time I was allowed raisins or a banana, while my brother helped himself to any food in the house.

I, on the other hand, began to hide and sneak my food. The frozen cupcakes in the freezer (which must have been for the other members of our household, because I was never handed one) the cookies, cans of cold raviolis and on some desperate occasions the frosting my mom stored for making cakes became my friend. Although I scored countless achievements in dance, and school activities, nothing that I did felt as successful as the summer I lost 8 pounds. I was 12.

Even so, it seemed like I just never quite fit in. Not with

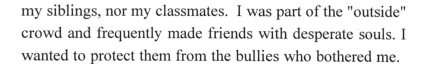

my siblings, nor my classmates. I was part of the "outside" crowd and frequently made friends with desperate souls. I wanted to protect them from the bullies who bothered me.

Carrying on through high school I was still chubby. Never really fitting in with the other girls who I danced with I hung more with the guys. My freshman year I weighed close to 180 lbs. At age 15 I had a grand-mal seizure and the Dr.'s dicovered I had epilepsy. I began taking heavy medication. Just one more thing to seperate me from the other kids. I had mono my senior year of high school and became so ill I could barely eat for 6 months. I was down to 145. My thinnest ever.

As soon as I was healthy I began to eat again, and I mean EAT. In the next two years I gained 50+ pounds. I moved away from home, and began anti-anxiety medication and gained another 20. I continued to gain until at 22 years old I was at 220 lbs. When I should have been dating, and experiencing my 20's , I was frumpy and fat. I had Social Anxiety Disorder, although I didn't know it at the time. I was afraid to go out and meet new people in fear that they wouldn't like me, or that I would have a seizure in front of them and scare them away (which happened in public when I was 18).

I moved to a community full of homosexual men, with some friends who I knew were true and where I knew I would be safe from my own physical appearance, because they weren't interested in me for that. For the first time in my life I felt accepted, wanted, and beautiful. Just for who I was. For the way I laughed, thought and dreamed. Some of those people led me to become who I am today.

After finally meeting my husband (who loved me and met me at my highest weight) and having three kids, I topped out at 254 pounds with a BMI of 43. My two closest friends had gastric bypass surgery, and I had decided to look into it, but I was turned down by my primary physician.. Two years passed and I had almost given up.

While playing with my son one day, he called me "mommy big butt" and I decided I would no longer live my live as an obese person. I decided "No" was not the answer I would accept! After I had a C-section delivery with my daughter in September of 2005, then an emergency gallbladder surgery in December of 2005, I went around my physician and found a surgeon on my own, Dr. Paul Cirangle. I had a Vertical Gastrectomy on January 18, 2006. I chose the Vertical Gastrectomy because there would be no malabsoption with this surgery.

There was no intestinal re-routing, so the recovery was faster. They also remove the unused portion of your stomach with this procedure, therefore removing the Grehlin, the hormone that produces hunger. I thought with my young children, who were 3,2 and 3 months at the time of my surgery, I needed to absorb as many vitamins from my food as possible.

I have lost 120+ lbs and hope to never find them again. Ending up at a size 4-6 with a BMI of 22 is something I never possibly imagined, or even knew I was worth.

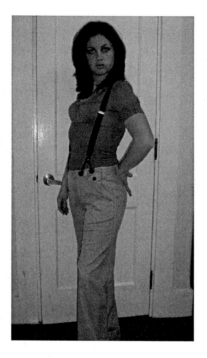

Deciding to have this surgery was life changing in so many ways it is difficult to choose where to start. As far as eating goes, I ate nothing but protein and vegetables for 6 months. I didn't snack unless absolutely necessary, and I got in my fluids EVERYDAY without exception. After 6 months I added in necessary carbs and actually had to up my calories as to not lose too much weight. I have a hard time with people who have had this surgery and complain about their lack of weight loss, yet they don't eat their protein or drink their fluids. I realize everyone is different, but to me, if I want to live a healthy successful life, these things are a must. Like Nike®, I just do it!

My husband is relentlessly supportive. He never gives up on me, and trusts that I am doing what is best for me and my family. He had no idea how things would turn out, and our relationship only gets stronger as time passes. I am very lucky to have someone so supportive in my corner. My parents knew I was having the surgery, and while they had valid concerns for their child, they supported me as well. They helped me through this as well.

I don't think my children remember me at my highest weight. They see pictures of me and sometimes do not know it is me. My three year old saw my wedding pictures (weighing 234 lbs) and he said "mom, you look all squished up!!". I will always treasure that description.

I attend a bariatric support group locally and it has helped me tremendously. I learn from other people's strengths and weakness. It keeps me on track when I am having a lack of will, and keeps me feeling supported, and never ever alone. These people are right there to support me whenever I need them, as well as amazing moderators who have been in our shoes. They are real people who continue to make mistakes, and move past them.

It's hard to believe that this is only the beginning of my story. I am looking towards the future filled with the ability to feel, love, think, dream and be.

TAKE THE
SUCCESS HABITS™ CHALLENGE!

Avoiding Grazing

1. Take inventory right now of what sort of snack foods you have around you. Are you surrounded with sweets? Chips and crackers? Identify what you have readily available and how it got there. Think of ways to make better choices.

2. Find and stock up on a good protein snack that you can carry with you for those times when you need something. Try jerky, a new cheese stick flavor, a Go-Gurt®, snap peas, etc.

3. Identify what the triggers are that cause you to graze. Is it a certain time of day, a certain place or activity? Be aware and plan ahead for those times and circumstances. Knowing is half the battle.

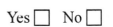

Success Habits™Principle 2
Portion Control

DAILY CHECK-UP QUESTIONS

I have eaten the proper quantity for
my stomach size at each meal.   Yes ☐   No ☐

I have eaten three meals today,
taking 20 to 30 minutes to eat.   Yes ☐   No ☐

I have eaten only what I planned
to eat today.   Yes ☐   No ☐

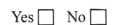

Success Habits™ Principle 3

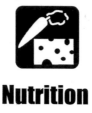

Nutrition

"I make good healthy food choices each day."

In this chapter we will briefly review some important things for weight-loss surgery patients to know about nutrition. I am not a dietician or a nutritionist and do not in any way intend to provide you with the many details you should know about your particular nutritional needs. This discussion is simply a compilation of a few basic principles.

First, you can imagine just how critically important it is to eat good food when you have a stomach the size of an egg. There is no room for junk! You must eat the most nutrient-dense foods possible.

While dietary guidelines differ, one thing I have found to be a common teaching among bariatric professionals is the need for protein. Many surgeons advocate 70 percent protein, 30 percent vegetables and NO refined carbohydrates. That means no bread, no pasta, no rice, no cookies, no candies, or cakes. No carbs! Been there, done that, you say? Well, perhaps, but the key difference here is that if you learn to fill up on protein first, it will take the edge off of your desire for the bread or pasta. Eat protein first, always and forever. I believe in this important principle, but it has not been an easy habit to acquire. I travel and eat out often. When dining out, what is the first thing they bring to your table when you sit down? Warm bread, rolls, or chips. I have learned to wait, eat protein first, then vegetables and then I will consider the carbohydrates if I am still hungry and most often I am not. Eating protein first is a habit that will serve you well your entire life. During your rapid weight-loss phase I encourage you to eat 70 percent protein and 30 percent vegetables, but after you have reached your goal weight you will be able to add some carbohydrate favorites. Once your goal weight is reached, BSCI's recommendation for your long-term weight maintenance is 50% protein, 25-30% carbohydrates and 20% - 25% fat. (Reference: BSCI's Maintenance Mentality by Janean G. Hall.)

I eat quite normally now but I am committed to eating protein first and then, if I am still hungry, I'll add a small portion of a carbohydrate or two.

In the following sections we will take a brief look at proteins, vegetables, carbohydrates, and fat.

THE POWER OF PROTEIN

Protein is essential for our good health. Our body digests protein more slowly than it does other foods and protein stays in our system longer, providing us with more consistent blood sugar levels.

The small stomach pouch of a weight-loss surgery patient has such a limited capacity, that in order to consume adequate amounts of protein each day, patients must maintain a diet consisting primarily of protein. Throughout the initial weight-loss phase, it is recommended that 70 percent of your diet should be protein. You must take responsibility to ensure that your body's protein stores are replenished each day.

There are two types of protein; those that contain all of the essential amino acids and those that do not. Nutritionists use the terms "complete protein" and "incomplete protein" to describe the differences found in various foods.

COMPLETE PROTEINS are derived from animal proteins, such as meat, chicken, eggs, fish, cheese and other milk products.

Grains and legumes, tofu and soy are also good sources of protein but do not, individually, have all of the essential amino acids and therefore are considered INCOMPLETE PROTEINS. Used together, such proteins can complement one another to form a complete protein.

Some foods that are great sources of protein are not good selections because they are too high in fat for those who struggle with their weight. Good selections include fish, poultry, low-fat cheeses, and low-fat milk. Proteins to use sparingly include beef, eggs (with yolk), whole milk, beans, legumes, and nuts.

TAKE THE
SUCCESS HABITS™ CHALLENGE!

Protein

1. Try a new protein. Something that you have never tried before or have not tried in a long time. How about tofu? Or soy? Or even liver! Then tell someone about it!

2. Find a new recipe for your favorite protein. Look for one in weight-loss surgery patient cookbooks or online at www.bariatricsupportcenter.com. See the section on Helpful People, Products and Programs

3. Stock up on your favorite protein snacks. Jerky, string cheese, Go-gurt®, etc. Find something you enjoy and make sure you keep a good supply on hand for those times when you need a little something.

In the next section we will discuss more about the importance of making high protein and low fat food choices.

THE VALUE OF VEGETABLES

A vegetable is defined as: any plant with edible parts, especially leafy or fleshy parts that are used mainly for soups and salads and to accompany main courses. (Encarta Dictionary)

Thirty percent of a weight-loss surgery patient's diet should come from vegetables. Simply, that's two or three bites of protein to one bite of vegetables. Vegetables are an important and essential source of vitamins, minerals, and fiber, which are low in fat and calories. Here are a few examples of vitamins derived from vegetables.

VITAMIN A

Vitamin A is important for vision and healthy skin. Good sources of Vitamin A are tomatoes and tomato products, dark green leafy vegetables like spinach and turnip greens and orange-colored vegetables like carrots, sweet potatoes and pumpkin.

VITAMIN C

Vitamin C is necessary for healthy bones and teeth. Tomatoes, peppers, cabbage, potatoes and dark, leafy greens such as spinach, romaine lettuce and watercress are all good sources of Vitamin C.

CALCIUM

Calcium is required to maintain strong bones and is an essential part of a healthy diet. Good sources of calcium include cheese, yogurt and dark green leafy vegetables like broccoli and spinach.

POTASSIUM

Potassium is critical for maintaining a normal heart rhythm and mineral balance. Cooked greens like spinach, baked sweet potato and winter squash are good sources of potassium.

TIP: If you are struggling to get your vegetables in each day try V-8 or other vegetable juice.

UNDERSTANDING CARBOHYDRATES

During the weight-loss phase following weight-loss surgery, patients are encouraged to eat 70 percent protein and 30 percent vegetables and eliminate most carbohydrates from their diet (specifically, bread, pasta, rice, potatoes, chips, cookies, candy, cakes, etc.). In doing so, the body is encouraged to utilize its fat stores for energy.

When carbohydrates are consumed, the body breaks them down into sugar glucose. Glucose is necessary to help maintain tissue protein, metabolize fat, and provide fuel for the central nervous system. Glucose is absorbed through the intestinal wall. If it is not utilized, it is stored in the liver and muscles as glycogen or in the fat cells as fat.

This leftover glucose is stored in your liver and muscles, and it's called glycogen.

The glycogen that doesn't fit into your liver and muscle cells is turned to fat.

Carbohydrates are classified into two categories: complex carbohydrates and refined carbohydrates.

Complex carbohydrates molecular complexity requires our bodies to work to break them down into a simpler form. Vegetables are complex carbohydrates and are an important source of energy.

Refined carbohydrates, known also as simple sugars, require little digestion and are too quickly absorbed, triggering the release of the hormone insulin. This causes a

TAKE THE
SUCCESS HABITS™ CHALLENGE!

Vegetables

1. Try a new vegetable; something that you have never tried before or have not tried in a long time. How about snap peas? Or Jicama? Good stuff!

2. Find a new recipe for your favorite vegetable. Share it with others at support group or post it online. See our section on Helpful People, Programs, and Products. Enjoy!

3. Take a class or check out a book on vegetable carvings. Learn how to make fancy food displays from all sorts of vegetables like a rose radish or fun vegetable animals. Share your talent with others or do it just for the fun of it.

rapid rise and subsequent fall of blood sugar levels. Refined carbohydrates usually come with lots of fat and very few vitamins.

Eliminating all carbohydrates, except vegetables, is important during the initial weight-loss phase or at any time when weight loss is desired. Once you've reached your goal weight, all types of carbohydrates can be slowly introduced back into the diet, in moderation. As long as weight is maintained, carbohydrates can be a great addition to provide variety and taste. But, if pounds start to creep back on, refined carbohydrates must be the first to go.

THE SKINNY ON FAT

Through many years of fighting the weight-loss battle, we have come to see fat as Enemy Number 1, and it certainly can be if we do not understand how our body burns or stores it. As weight-loss surgery patients, we need to regulate how much fat we have in our diets because the amount changes a great deal throughout the first year or so following surgery.

New patients (up to 6 months after surgery) need not worry as much about the percentage of fat in the foods they consume as patients whose surgery was a year or more previous. So, early on, it isn't necessary to be overly concerned about the fat content in the foods you eat. In time, however, as your stomach capacity increases, it will become increasingly important to pay attention to the fat content in your food choices.

Peanuts are a source of protein. A few, an ounce or two, probably won't hurt you and may give you a good energy boost. Early on, you might be satisfied with just a few. But, if that few turns into a cupful of this high-fat protein source, you may be in trouble. Fat, in a limited quantity is important for our bodies. It is important to understand how your body metabolizes fat, why you need it and how you can teach your body to burn it!

The body requires some fat to maintain good health. Things such as a strong immune system, healthy skin and hair and the ability to clot blood normally all depend on sufficient fat stores within the body.

Proteins end up as amino acids in the blood. Carbohydrates turn into blood glucose. The fat we consume, however, ends up as high and low density cholesterol, monoglycerides, triglycerides and fatty acids.

Fatty acids are small and very mobile within our systems. They move in and out of the blood stream in search of muscle cells in need of fuel to be burned as energy.

If we do not use fatty acids for fuel, we store them in fat depots throughout our bodies. Once stored as triglycerides, they must be disassembled back into fatty acids in order for them to be burned as fuel.

To reduce our fat stores, we must first stop filling them up with unused fatty acids and then we need to exercise in order to burn what has already been stored.

Recently, after having gained a few unwanted pounds, I took a very close look at the things that I was eating and drinking on a regular basis. I found that there were many things in my diet that were there, not because I liked them, but because eating them had become a mindless habit. I realized that I was making some poor choices at the grocery store, again out of habit. I decided to pay attention! As I began our Back on Track Program, I began to pay very close attention to not only the protein that has always been a priority, but the total carbohydrates, fat and calories that I was consuming. As many do, I found that I was consuming far more calories than I needed from several things that really did not matter to me. And most of the excess calories were coming from fat. For instance, I do not like milk- at all. So why then would I buy whole milk or 2% or even 1% milk to cook with and such, when skim would be fine?

I also recognized that I am so tired of having to think about right foods, wrong foods, this brand, that brand, this type of fat, that type of fat, good carbs, bad carbs!! It all becomes overwhelming, confusing and time consuming. My husband and I decided to do our homework, research the foods we were purchasing, and make a decision once and for all as to what we would buy and which brands we liked that also fit our budget. We researched, shopped and compared and made our shopping decisions. Thank goodness, we won't have to re-think that ever again! We have made some good new choices that surprisingly, add up to quite a difference.

By mindfully shopping and making our selections ON PURPOSE, (instead of the usual grab the cheapest and go) we effectively cut out hundreds of calories. Fat filled calories hidden in foods that simply DO NOT MATTER!

Here is our list of the changes we have made:

2 Eggs only 1 yolk instead of 2 eggs	SAVINGS 40 calories
Skim Milk instead of 2%	SAVINGS 30 calories
Light dressing instead of regular	SAVINGS 30 calories
Light mayonnaise instead of regular	SAVNGS 30 calories
Water with lime instead of Fitness Water	SAVINGS 30 calories
Fat free cottage cheese instead of 4%	SAVINGS 21 calories
An apple instead of a banana	SAVINGS 63 calories
Light margarine instead of regular	SAVINGS 40 calories

TOTAL SAVINGS OF 284 calories!!!!!

What a great lesson! As you can see most of the savings have come from cutting out the fat. May I encourage you to take some time read the labels on the foods you eat regularly and see where you might be able to save some calories.

TAKE THE
SUCCESS HABITS™ CHALLENGE!

Fat

1. Do some comparison shopping and note the fat content in different types of cheeses. Which cheese has the most fat? Which cheese has the least amount of fat? Give a new type of cheese a try.

2. Try a new type of milk. If you are using whole milk, switch to 2 percent; if you are using 2 percent, switch to 1 percent; if 1 percent, try skim.

3. Try a new "lite" way to cook your meat. On the BBQ, the broiler. Bake it or grill it, anything but fry it!

Success Habits™Principle 3
Nutrition

DAILY CHECK-UP QUESTIONS

✔

I ate 70 percent protein today. Yes ☐ No ☐

I ate 30 percent vegetables today. Yes ☐ No ☐

I avoided refined carbohydrates today. Yes ☐ No ☐

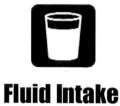

Fluid Intake

"I drink the right amount of the right beverages at the right time each day."

One of the most difficult, but essential habits to acquire is the habit of proper drinking. Experience has taught me that there are several key factors in learning to drink the right substances in the right quantity and at the right time. Throughout this chapter we will discuss several important drinking habits.

First, the "when." We'll learn about the importance of not drinking at the same time that we eat. Second, we'll learn about how and why our bodies need the proper amount of liquid each day and what beverages are recommended. Next, we'll take a look at some of the beverages thought to be harmful to weight-loss surgery patients.

EATING AND DRINKING AT THE SAME TIME

Weight-loss surgery patients are encouraged to avoid eating and drinking at the same time for one primary reason; our need for satiety. You see, if the name of the game is to feel full and satisfied on very little food, then you don't want to eat and drink at the same time or drink right after you eat, as it will flush the food through your system too quickly. The consequence: you feel hungry again sooner than you should. And many eat again too soon, resulting in greater calorie consumption than is actually needed and - you guessed it - weight gain.

Several years ago, a patient out four months from surgery came in to one of our classes and exclaimed, "I don't think they even did anything in there. I can eat four cheese sandwiches all at once!"

My first thought was, "Why are you eating cheese sandwiches?" and second, "How are you eating four cheese sandwiches?" Her weight loss was not where it should have been for four months post op and, of course, she was terribly discouraged. After some initial discussion we discovered how and why this was happening. She was eating a little and drinking a little, eating then drinking, eating then drinking. She was constantly forcing the food through the anastamosis into the intestine, then she felt hungry again right away and ate additional food to satisfy the hunger. Although this is a simple concept, you can see how easily this tool can be compromised. I am sure this woman was uncomfortable and yet she continued to eat and drink, eat and drink and as a result, she ate far more than her body needed. Once again, having a small stomach pouch is a tool that can serve you well your entire life, but you must learn to use it properly. One of the primary benefits to having weight-loss surgery is that we are able to stay full and satisfied on very little food. To maintain that full feeling, we must not eat and drink at the same time. My doctor recommended that I wait at least 30 minutes after eating before I resume drinking again. There are a number of other bariatric surgeons who encourage their patients to wait for over an hour after eating. I have found that waiting 30 minutes or so has worked well for me, but understanding your body's tendencies can help you identify what's best for you. Start by doing a little experiment to see if you can determine how drinking affects both the quantity of food you are able to eat and the length of time you are able to stay full. Next, study the results of your experiment to determine the ideal length of time between eating and drinking for your body.

COFFEES AND TEAS

With a small, newly created stomach pouch, it is essential to avoid any harmful substance that could cause ulcers or inflict damage to the stomach, namely, coffees and teas. While we know that some patients return to drinking these beverages through the years, experience has shown that most successful patients do not. This, in my mind, has been enough to convince me that this is an important habit for success. Here are several reasons for the cautionary measures regarding these beverages.

CAFFEINE

Coffees and Teas contain a significant amount of caffeine. A study by researchers at Duke University Medical Center, [reported in the Duke Medical News], shows that caffeine taken in the morning has effects on the body that persist until bedtime and amplifies stress consistently throughout the day. These results show for the first time that the effects of caffeine last considerably longer than originally thought . . . and that caffeine exaggerates stress in people who consume it every day. When the researchers compared the caffeine days to the placebo days they discovered that caffeine consumption significantly raised systolic and diastolic blood pressure consistently throughout the day and night, and adrenaline levels rose by 32 percent. The researchers found that the elevated levels persisted as the evening progressed to bedtime. The study, which was funded by the National Institutes of Health, appears in the July/August 2002 issue of Psychosomatic Medicine.

"The effects of coffee drinking are long-lasting and exaggerate the stress response both in terms of the body's physiological response in blood pressure elevations and stress hormone levels, but it also magnifies a person's perception of stress," said James D. Lane, Ph.D., associate research professor in the department of psychiatry and behavioral sciences at Duke and lead author of the study. "People haven't really accepted the fact that there could be a health downside to caffeine consumption, but our evidence - and that of other studies - shows that this downside exists and people should be aware of it in order to make the best possible health choices."

The study also showed that while caffeine increases blood pressure and heart rate, it also amplifies those effects at the times when participants report higher levels of stress during their day. The caffeine appears to compound the effects of stress both psychologically in terms of perceived stress levels and physiologically in terms of elevated blood pressures and stress hormone levels - as if the stressor is actually of greater magnitude, he said.

"The caffeine we drink enhances the effects of the stresses we experience, so if we have a stressful job, drinking coffee makes our body respond more to the ordinary stresses we experience," he said. "The combination of stress and caffeine has a multiplying, or synergistically negative effect.

"Everyone accepts that stress can be unhealthy. Our results suggest that drinking coffee or other caffeinated drinks can make stress even more unhealthy." Increased stress is known to contribute to unhealthy eating habits in obese individuals. Caffeine is also a stimulant and has been known to increase hunger. Increased hunger is, of course, detrimental to weight loss and long-term weight control.

TAKE THE
SUCCESS HABITS™ CHALLENGE!

Caffeine

1. Learn more about the effects of caffeine by reading books, magazine articles, and online resourses.

2. Give herbals a chance. Try one or more of the many flavors that are available in herbal teas. Other hot drinks that you may enjoy include broth, spiced cider, and so on.

CALCIUM LOSS

Many believe that caffeine contributes to osteoporosis or calcium loss in women. In its January 1994 edition, pages 280-283, the Journal of the American Medical Association states, "There was a significant association between drinking more caffeinated coffee and decreasing bone mineral density at both the hip and the spine, independent of age, obesity, years since menopause and the use of tobacco, estrogen, alcohol, thiazides and calcium supplements in women."

It is critically important for weight-loss surgery patients to take extra caution to avoid consuming anything that would be detrimental to the new stomach pouch.

As weight-loss surgery patients, we must not consume anything that would limit our already limited capacity to absorb essential vitamins and nutrients.

If you enjoy herbal teas, by all means, make them as part of your beverage choices. Again, we are encouraged to select a variety of beverages to meet our daily fluid quota of sixty-four ounces.

For many, coffee and tea have become a very routine part of the day and giving them up can be quite difficult, especially when these beverages contain caffeine. Some quitters have found it helpful to cut down their intake by 1/2 cup each day, while others choose to quit "cold turkey".

Withdrawal symptoms from reducing caffeine intake can be significant, such as nervousness, restlessness, irritability and headaches. These symptoms can be countered with exercise, sleep and by replacing these beverages with healthier alternatives.

ALCOHOL

As a rule, weight-loss surgery patients should use great caution when it comes to alcoholic beverages. There are a number of reasons for this. First, alcoholic beverages are often high in calories. Excess calories can easily be consumed by drinking them without thinking. A second reason for additional caution is that many alcoholic beverages are carbonated and carbonation should be avoided. The third and primary concern is the rapid rate of absorption in weight-loss surgery patients. Weight-loss surgery allows for food and drink to be absorbed very quickly into the bloodstream. This raises several questions:

- Do weight-loss surgery patients absorb things differently than "normal" people?

- Can weight-loss surgery patients get drunk more quickly than "normal" people?

- Can weight-loss surgery patients get drunk on less alcohol than "normal" people?

To increase my understanding of the effects of alcohol on a weight-loss surgery patient, I consulted with the bariatric surgeons from Rocky Mountain Associated Physicians in Salt Lake City, Utah. They provided me with the following consensus statement: "Patients are cautioned with respect to alcohol consumption after Roux-en-Y weight-loss surgery (RNYGBP). Studies have shown that alcohol absorption is more rapid following RNYGBP."

A weight-loss surgery patient may become intoxicated with lesser amounts of alcohol than a normal person may. However, intoxication is determined by blood alcohol levels. The intoxication level of blood alcohol is the same in a weight-loss surgery patient as it is in any other person."

It is important for weight loss surgery patients to also use great caution when using over the counter cold medicines and cough syrups, which contain a high concentration of alcohol.

Recently, the issue of transfer addiction in WLS patients has caught the media's attention. Are WLS patients more susceptible to transferring their addiction for food to alcohol? Perhaps. There are no definitive answers at this point, but the interest has sparked a number of bariatric researchers to begin to investigate.

Key points to remember:
- Weight-loss surgery patients can become intoxicated on less alcohol.

- Weight-loss surgery patients can become intoxicated more quickly than others.

- Blood alcohol level is blood alcohol level regardless of how much is consumed or over what period of time. In essence, drunk is drunk!

Weight-loss surgery patients should also be wary of over-the-counter and prescription cold and/or cough medicines, which often contain high concentrations of alcohol.

THE IMPORTANCE OF WATER

Water is our very essence. It is the most important nutrient in our body. Water makes up 70 percent of our muscles and 75 percent of our brain. The only thing that our bodies crave more than water is oxygen.

Water helps us maintain proper muscle tone, prevents dehydration, improves our skin and hair, and helps rid the body of waste and harmful toxins. It increases our energy level, suppresses our appetite, and helps to maintain our weight. It is absolutely essential to our good health and well-being.

TAKE THE
SUCCESS HABITS™ CHALLENGE!

Avoiding Alcohol

1. Take a moment to read the labels on all of the cold or cough syrups you may have. Be sure you have a non-alcoholic type of medicine for your needs.

Drinking enough water is a challenge for many, but for some, drinking water at all is a chore. It is a common sight these days to see people carrying bottled or filtered water with them. There are countless reasons for this, including:

The taste of bottled or filtered water is preferred over the taste of tap water.

Bottled water offers consumers added convenience, including the option to fill and refill the bottles.

Many prefer ice-cold water and find freezing their bottled water overnight provides them with cold water throughout the following day.

And still others seek water of a higher quality.

THE GOOD, THE BAD AND THE TOXIC!

Water quality is certainly a concern in most cities. SELF magazine in August 1997 featured an article entitled, "Is Your Drinking Water Safe?" They stated that, "Approximately 50 million Americans, roughly one in five, are exposed to potentially harmful levels of hazardous materials whenever they open their faucet."

Additionally, the July 18, 2000, edition of the New York Times reported that "The concern about water safety has prompted millions of Americans to reject the water that comes straight from the tap, resulting in two new growth industries: bottled water and filtration systems."

Because, as weight-loss surgery patients, we do not drink while we eat, we must be ever-mindful of the need to drink between meals. This requires planning, discipline and formation of a new habit. I have never been a "soda pop" drinker. I have always considered myself a good water drinker but it was not until I started measuring that I realized that while I thought I was getting enough, I was no where near the recommended 64 ounces per day.

I have been very happy with my decision a few years ago to purchase a special portable filtered water bottle. It is designed to filter out the contaminants and restore the water to its natural "living" state. I know what's in it, I know what isn't, and I know how much I am drinking each day. I have a carrying case which has made it easy to have my water with me constantly, and regardless of the source, the water tastes the same. Although purchasing a quality filtered water bottle was an investment, it has been well worth the cost because I am a much better water drinker and I'm convinced that it is essential for my good health.

THE DANGERS AND SIGNS OF DEHYDRATION:

Throughout the day, the average adult can lose up to eight to ten cups of water through regular activities, evapo-

TAKE THE
SUCCESS HABITS™ CHALLENGE!

The Dangers of Dehydration

1. Begin each day this week by pre-measuring the 64 ounces of beverage(s) you will drink that day. See how close you come to your quota.

2. Try a new beverage. How about an herbal tea, or a flavored water? Or, simply add a slice of lemon or lime to your water. And don't forget all of those great vegetable juices.

3. Shop for a new container to carry your beverage with you. There are many types of sports bottles, insulated mugs, carriers, etc.

ration, exhaling and urinating. Eight to ten cups! And that is before doing any sort of strenuous exercise.

When we fail to replenish our bodies' losses each day, dehydration becomes a threat to our health. Dehydration is defined as the condition in which the body suffers from lack of water and blood salts. The kidneys, heart, brain and other vital organs must have the proper amounts of water and salt in order to function properly.

New weight-loss surgery patients must be especially careful to avoid dehydration during the early stages following surgery. The signs of dehydration are as follows:

Mild Dehydration: Thirst, Dry Lips, Dry Mouth

Moderate Dehydration: Very dry mouth, sunken
    eyes, skin that doesn't bounce back to the touch.

Severe Dehydration: All signs of moderate dehydration
    plus weak pulse, cold hands and feet, rapid
    breathing, blue lips, confusion, lethargy and
    difficulty arousing.

While mild and moderate dehydration can be self-treated, severe dehydration should be treated by a medical professional. IV therapy may be used to restore fluids quickly and can be life-saving.

To prevent dehydration, experts recommend that people drink at least 64 ounces (6 to 8 glasses) of water each day. The recommended drinking water quotient takes into account the 3 to 4 ounces typically consumed through foods like fruits and vegetables, which are about 80 percent water. Although 6 to 8 glasses is the standard recommendation for the typical adult, weight-loss surgery patients must be sure to get at least that much each day. This can be quite a challenge for new weight-loss surgery patients, who often take several months to work up to the recommended 64 ounces.

THE DANGERS OF CARBONATION

One of the most controversial issues among weight-loss surgery patients is whether or not drinking carbonated beverages is detrimental to them. Does it hinder weight loss? Cause weight gain? Stretch the stomach pouch? Ruin the anastamosis? What do we know about the answers to these important questions? What have our years of experience with patients taught us about the effects of drinking carbonation?

Weight-loss surgery patients who are most successful in reaching and maintaining their goal weight do not drink carbonated beverages. We have also observed time and time again, that those who have regained a significant amount of weight and have come back to us have usually gone back to drinking carbonated beverages. These two findings point out that avoiding carbonated drinks is an important habit for our long-term success.

There are three primary reasons to avoid carbonated beverages, as per Dr. Charles Edwards:

1. Distention of the stomach pouch and anastamosis:

When a cold, carbonated beverage is consumed, it warms and releases gases, distending (expanding) the stomach pouch. This stretching of the stomach then creates undue stress and, subsequently, may cause stretching of the anastamosis. It is important for this "outlet" (the anastamosis) to stay small and tight in order for the food to empty slowly from the stomach pouch. If it is stretched, the ability to feel full is compromised, and overeating is usually the result.

2. Caloric Intake:

Many carbonated beverages are high in calories, lowin nutritional value and contain simple sugars. Not only do they add additional calories with low nutritional value, they are absorbed quickly into the blood stream, sometimes causing a rapid rise in blood sugar, elevated insulin levels, and increased hunger.

3. Caffeine:

Many carbonated beverages contain caffeine, which many believe to be an appetite stimulant, which is detrimental to initial weight loss and long-term weight maintenance.

Fortunately, I have never been one to drink carbonated beverages and so this was not a challenge for me, but it is for many. Through the years I have worked with thousands of weight-loss surgery patients, the majority of which are former soda-pop drinkers. And believe me, I have heard it all. One gentleman said that he simply could not give up his Diet Coke, so he purchased a gallon of the syrup to add to his water! Others call and ask, "I have had my soda in the microwave for an hour to take out the carbonation, can I drink it now?" And many comment that they simply open the can or bottle and let their pop go flat for several days before drinking it. To them I say, "Whatever!"

Giving up carbonated beverages is an important habit which will undoubtedly require commitment, determination and self control. This lifestyle change will be one that will improve your weight loss and maintenance as well as your overall health and well-being.

Patients who participate in our programs are counseled prior to surgery on all of the Success Habits™ principles. Many who struggle with the idea of giving up their diet sodas choose to stop drinking them a month or two before surgery. Some have shared that they wanted to be sure that they could do it. Others do so to get a head start on their new habits. And still others have wanted to give them up for many years.

While there are many stories of people who struggle in their efforts to give up carbonated beverages, there are thousands more who have forsaken them and are happier and healthier as a result. Here is one such story.

Pamm's Story

I have been heavy my entire life, but by the time my weight reached 305 pounds, my life was exhausting and embarrassing. I just existed day to day, not living life the way it is meant to be lived.

My day would start with a walk to the refrigerator to pour myself a Pepsi. I was a Pepsi-aholic. I drank six to eight cans of Pepsi a day, depending on my stress level. Pepsi was to me like a cigarette is to a smoker. I could not go anywhere without a Pepsi in my hand. My husband would tease me about putting an intravenous line of Pepsi into my arm to help me throughout the day. If Pepsi had a poster child, it would have been me.

At 305 pounds I was continually tired, even when I just woke up. I teach third grade, which is not an easy job. I found myself having to sit throughout the day while I taught, instead of walking around and helping the students.

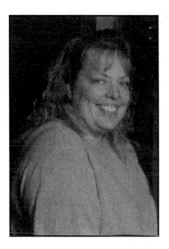

They would have to come to my desk in order for me to help them with any problems. When I first began teaching I would walk around the classroom while reading to the students, but with my heavy weight I would have to sit at my desk.

After school I would be so tired that I had to go home and take a nap. My own children saw the importance of their mom getting a nap. If someone was to call or come and visit they would tell him or her that I was busy or unavailable to see them. The last thing I wanted people to know was that my weight was causing me problems.

My weight was taking away any hope of a quality life. I couldn't do any physical things with my children such as hiking, biking, jumping on the trampoline, hide-and-go-seek, or even going for a walk. I was constantly too tired for any physical activities.

Other simple things were a chore, like getting out of my car when I would pick my son up from school. I would either honk my horn or send my daughter in to get him. I was just too tired to pick myself up after teaching all day.

Even housework was a challenge for me. If I put in a load of laundry and changed it to the dryer, it wasn't too bad because I could rest in between. However, when it came time to unload the dryer and then carry the basket, I would have to wait until the next day to fold the clothes and put them away.

The concerning time in my life came when my doctor told me that I was going to die if I didn't make a change in my weight situation. When you weigh 305 pounds it is not as easy as it sounds. I told my doctor of my fears of dying and not knowing how to make a change because I had tried everything else that I thought was available. My doctor recommended that I have the weight-loss surgery and stated that it would work. I finally felt some peace of mind. I made an appointment with a surgeon for June 1, 2001. I truly felt like I would finally get the help I needed. I went to my appointment and found out I more than qualified for the surgery.

I was so thrilled! I finally felt like I had a chance. I attended the Surgical Solution™ Presentation presented by Bariatric Support Centers International, only to find out that my insurance would not cover me financially for the procedure. My disappointment cannot be expressed in words. I knew that I needed the surgery. I decided I would visit the insurance company with letters from several doctors stating the necessity of the surgery; that it was not just a way to lose weight but rather a life-or-death situation.

I was hoping that putting a face with the request would help persuade them to cover the procedure. I just knew that they would see my situation and understand why I had to have this surgery. I explained how I would need two knee surgeries along with a hip replacement and the risks of diabetes and heart disease if I didn't get the weight off.

The insurance company stated that they would gladly pay for the knee and hip replacements but refused to cover the bypass surgery. The woman reached across the desk, took my hand, and asked in a soft tone, "Honey, have you tried Weight Watchers?" At that point I began to cry. I knew that I was destined to be heavy, unhealthy, and pretty much miserable for the rest of my life. Driving home, all I could do was cry; I feared that all I could do was somehow make the change on my own. I tried walking up and down the block in front of my house, but was unable to even make it to a few houses down the street. I was so out of breath and tired I thought I was going to die.

In the last week of June, I was taking my third-grade class on a walking field trip. We were going to be walking for one mile. I was very nervous because waking was so difficult for me. I thought, in the back of my mind, that I would be all right because the beginning of the trip was all down hill, but I was extremely worried about the return trip. My teammates knew of my concerns and let me lead us back so I could set the pace. Even with this accommodation, when we started up the hill, I knew I was in trouble.

About halfway up the hill, I was huffing and puffing so badly my students began to worry. They kept asking if I was okay because they began to see how tired I was getting and how red my face began to get. 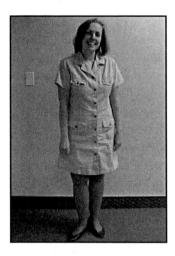 It got to the point where I couldn't even answer them because I was so out of breath. Finally I had to stop and rest. I was beginning to wonder if I was going to be able to make it back up the hill. After a long rest I was able to make it to the top of the hill but not without a lot of shortness of breath and exhaustion. After much concern from the students and my teammates, we sat down for another long rest. The whole time I just kept thinking, "Once I get back to school, I can just sit down and I will be okay."

I will never forget how awful that walk was for me. I did finally make it back to school, but I was sick and hurting. After school I went straight home and went to bed.

This was the turning point in my life. I knew I had to find funding for the surgery. The next step was finding the courage to ask my father for a loan, which was a very hard thing for me to do. I went to my dad and explained my situation and my fears. He said that he just didn't feel right about paying that much money for weight loss. I was devastated. I felt that he was my last hope.

Three months went by, and my father sold his home and moved in with my family and me. This was an eye-opening experience for my dad. Now he witnessed first-hand how much my weight had affected my life and my health. After seeing my daily activities for two days, he came to me and told me that after seeing my situation, he would gladly lend me the money to help with the medical costs.

I can't tell you the relief and happiness that overcame me at that moment. The next morning I called my surgeon and scheduled surgery for December 13, 2001, at 10:00 a.m. On that day, I was reborn. I was able to begin my life again and be healthy. I sincerely feel that weight-loss surgery has saved my life and have never regretted making the decision. Since the surgery I have followed my doctor's counsel and have maintained a steady weight-loss. Despite the complications I had following surgery, I would make the same decision to have surgery again without hesitation. The classes and weigh-ins provided by the Bariatric Support Center have beed extremely helpful for me. By following the six Success Habits™ principles, I have been extremely successful. I have lost 150 pounds and I am living my life to its fullest. I exercise every morning, play with my children, swim, hike, bike, and do so many activities that I couldn't do before. My energy level has increased tremendously and I now feel like there is nothing that I can't do. What a dramatic difference from just one year ago!"

TAKE THE
SUCCESS HABITS™ CHALLENGE!

Avoiding Carbonation

1. To learn more about carbonation, do one of the following experiments:

Supplies Needed: One cold can of a diet soda and one quart plastic bag with a sealable opening –OR– One cold bottle of diet soda and one balloon

Open the cold can of pop and pour rapidly into the sealable plastic bag, which represents your stomach pouch. Toss it around a bit, and then simply let it sit for a while. As the carbonated beverage warms up it will release gas and will bloat and distend the bag. Leave it for several days and you will note how long the the carbonation stays in the bag! –OR– Open and place the balloon over a cold bottle of soda pop. Shake a bit and watch it blow up the balloon as time goes on.

2. Give it up! Find a replacement. As we have learned in our study of habit change, it is necessary for long-term success to replace an old habit with a new one. Find something new to drink, flavored water, or diet juice drinks.

Success Habits™ Principle 4
Fluid Intake

DAILY CHECK-UP QUESTIONS

✔

I drink at least 64 ounces of fluid daily. Yes ☐ No ☐

I do not drink carbonated beverages. Yes ☐ No ☐

I do not eat and drink together. Yes ☐ No ☐

By now the drink of choice for weight-loss surgery patients has likely become painfully obvious to you. You've read about the importance of avoiding carbonation, coffee, tea and alcohol. What does that leave? Yes, you've got it!   Water.

Success Habits™ Principle 5

Regular Exercise

"I have adopted the habit of exercise
as part of my lifestyle."

On the northwest corner wall of the gym where I exercise hangs a large poster in a plastic frame. It features success stories of gym clients with before and after pictures and a few quotes. When I first saw the poster, I read the inspiring stories and oohed and aahed at the pictures, but it wasn't too long before I stopped paying much attention to it. The poster just became part of the wall that I ignored even though my morning circuit training routine takes me into that particular corner three different times.

Then one day, one memorable day when the lighting was just right, I happened to actually look at the poster again and could see my reflection in the warped plastic frame. What I saw horrified me. In the reflection I appeared to be my true height of 5 feet, 2 inches, only I was twice as wide! I still shudder when I think about that awful sight!

In that instant my thoughts turned to how I had looked seven years earlier when I weighed 250 pounds. The memory of myself as a fat woman is etched clearly in my mind and with it comes all the heartache and all the pain that I felt as a result of my weight. It was very hard for me to stand there in that gym and face my former self. Doing so brought back some ugly memories and sensitive feelings. But, it served as an important reminder of where I have been and where I could find myself again if I'm not diligent in my efforts.

Several weeks after my little experience with the reflection, I found myself in the same corner of the same gym, only this time I was facing the opposite direction. The blinds were up and it was still dark outside. Once again, the lighting was just right for me to see my reflection. As I looked in the window, I thought, hey, that's me; kind of a cute little thing all dressed in my workout sweats! And then an interesting thought came to mind. Here I stand: before me my true reflection, behind me the distorted one; and I can choose to face either way. Which direction are you facing? It's OK to reflect on the past, but always look to the future.

REGULAR EXERCISE

Often I hear the question, "If I was able to commit to eating right and exercising, why would I need surgery?" If I have not been disciplined enough in the past, what makes you think that I will be able to commit to this in the future?"

My response is inevitably, "Well, that is up to you. The decision to have surgery or not is up to you. The decision to comply with the guidelines or not is up to you, whether or not you believe in and internalize these Success Habits™ principles is up to you."

"I know, I know," they respond, "but do I have to exercise?"

"Yes, you must exercise!" is always my response. We do have patients who do not exercise, this is true, but our most successful long-term patients use exercise as a tool to help control their weight. From them I hear comments such as, "I lead a very normal life now. I eat normally; the main difference is that now I exercise. If I find myself regaining, I add a few minutes each session, or add another session each week, but exercise is a key factor in controlling my weight."

This is one of the most important lessons that I have learned from the successful patients who have gone before me. The message from them is clear: exercise is critical to maintaining the balance between Calories-In and Calories-Out. As much as we all would like to believe that exercise is not an essential habit to our long-term success, it is! And therefore, we must! I do, do you?

Throughout the years I have been, let's say, a fair exerciser. I have experimented with just about every type of exercise, every time of day and every game or gimmick that I could find to keep myself motivated to stick with it. I have joined gyms, workout studios, done lap swimming, water aerobics, circuit training, and oh, of course there was a time when I convinced myself that bowling was exercise! NOT!

As I look back through the years, I have come to recognize that the times when I was the most committed to exercising were the times when I was focused on losing weight. It was never for fun, never for good health. It was always a means to an end: weight loss. It was always about work, and rarely did I actually enjoy it. However, I did enjoy the boost to my self-esteem when I boasted to friends and family that I had been "working out" or that I was "at the gym." But, that immediate feeling of accomplishment was short-lived and certainly not enough of a reason to get up and go one more day. And so, many gym memberships expired, many aerobic classes continued on without me, and my weight continued to go up and down, up and down. Sound familiar?

It is easy to see now that while I was exercising, I was losing weight (duh!). But, once I went off whatever diet it was, I stopped exercising, the weight I'd lost returned and then some (double duh!) and it became increasingly difficult to give it another try. New diet, new exercise routine, some success, life happened, more failure. New diet, new exercise program, some success, life happened, more failure. The battle with myself to exercise soon became just a routine part of my war with my weight. And it was a war I was losing. As weight piled on, my interest in exercise decreased dramatically, my desire to even try just disappeared. But then . . .

Following my weight-loss surgery. I was losing weight and feeling better every day. I knew I needed to exercise and wanted to exercise but I was also all too familiar with pitfalls of time and circumstances that had been my challenges throughout the years. So I set out to eliminate any possible obstacle that would keep me from following through. I had to first deal with my many excuses to not exercise: the gym is too far away and I don't like to drive. I don't have the money, it's too cold outside, it's too hot outside, I don't like people watching me, I don't like the music they play, I don't like to haul my clothes, makeup, etc. to the gym, it's too hard, it's too easy, I don't like the instructor, I don't like the person next to me, it's too crowded, the class is at the wrong time, the aerobic rider downstairs hurts my back and it's too cold downstairs anyway! With all these well- founded excuses, I knew that I wouldn't get anywhere until I could figure out something that was "custom made" just for me. Here's what I did:

I had my husband make me an exercise tape of my favorite old rock 'n roll songs. Each morning after he went to work and and kids were off to school I would crank it up and dance, and exercise alone in my bedroom. I developed quite a routine! It was one that I enjoyed, not too hard, not too easy, and one customized just for me. No need to drive anywhere, no one to bother me, or see me, no cost, in my own time. I became an avid exerciser.

Now, not everyone shares the same challenges with the hassles of exercising that I do. But I suspect that each of you can identify with one or two of them. I'll bet that you have hang-ups of your own as well. So, what are they? What are the obstacles that are stopping you from exercising? May I encourage you to take some time to identify them? Write them down and then blow holes in them by doing whatever it takes to remove them. Then take some time to evaluate the reasons you exercise. Is it because you "have to?" Is it a social event for you? Is it to lose weight or for your health? Is it for your partner? As I have contemplated the many times I have stopped my exercise habit I have identified that my inconsistency and lack of stick-to-it-ive-ness were due to the reasons I was exercising in the first place.

To acquire a lifetime habit of exercise, I believe that these three motivating factors must be present:

1. *You must want to exercise for yourself and by yourself.*

2. *You must want to exercise for your health.*

3. *You must exercise because you enjoy it.*

So, what's it going to take?

JUST DO IT!

The most successful long-term patients are committed to exercise. Many of them comment that they are able to keep their weight in check simply through exercise. They report eating normally, enjoying a variety of foods, and also enjoying a more active lifestyle.

There are many common reasons people give for not exercising. No time, no energy, no money for equipment or gym memberships, etc. Whatever the reason or excuse, the trick is to "Get Over It," and "Just Do It!" Start today.

Here are some great motivational ideas to help you get moving!

• Pick a place on the map where you would like to travel that is approximately 1200 miles away. Chart your mileage. One minute of activity = 1 mile of travel towards your destination.

• Write down ten rewards on ten different slips of paper. Put them in a grab bag. Pick one slip of paper out of the grab bag each time you exercise. Do not reward yourself with food. Instead, use personal pampering things such as a manicure, a massage, new hair cut, etc.

> **"Regular exercise is important during weight-loss, but it is essential for long-term weight maintenance."**

• Set up an Activity Bank. Pay yourself $1 each day you have met your activity goal. Pay the bank each day you did

TAKE THE
***SUCCESS HABITS*™ CHALLENGE!**

Regular Exercise

1. What are the major obstacles that prevent you from exercising? List them on a piece of paper and analyze them one at a time. Are any of them insurmountable? Identify what has to happen for you to overcome them.

2. Make a call or a personal visit to a nearby gym, club or exercise studio. Investigate their programs, prices and match them to your needs and resources.

not. Treat yourself with a night out or a new outfit at the end of the month.

TARGET HEART RATE

Looking back I could see that as the years passed by and pounds piled on, exercise became less and less interesting and more and more difficult. Following weight-loss surgery, as weight drops and energy increases, exercise becomes easier, more appealing and even fun!

It is important to recognize that as a heavy person, you expended a great deal of energy just walking across the room. Any effort to exercise burned many calories. As your weight comes off and you become smaller, you must work harder to burn the same number of calories that you did as a larger person. Additionally, the more fit you become, the more diligent you must be in making sure that you are exercising in a manner that will provide you with optimal benefit.

In order to improve your cardiovascular fitness you must exercise hard enough to raise your heart rate, but not so hard that you over-exert. The American Heart Association advises people to exercise at 50 percent to 75 percent of their maximum heart rate. This is known as your Target Heart Rate, or THR. The following formula is an easy way to calculate your THR.

DETERMINING YOUR TARGET HEART RATE

1. Calculate your age predicted maximum heart rate

220 - _____ (age) = Age Predicted Heart Rate

2. Multiply your age predicted heart rate by 0.50:

_____ X 0.50 = _____

This is your lower heart rate limit for aerobic exercise

3. Multiply your age predicted heart rate by 0.75:

_____ X 0.75 = _____

This is your upper limit heart rate for aerobic exercise

4. Your Target Heart range is from _____ to _____

Now divide your rate by 6 for the number of beats per 10 second count

TAKE THE
SUCCESS HABITS™ CHALLENGE!

Target Heart Rate

1. Using the formula provided, calculate your target heart rate.

2. Begin a log to track your exercise workouts and your heart rate at the beginning, the middle, and the end of your routine.

EXERCISE FREQUENCY

The most successful long-term weight-loss surgery patients are maintaining their weight by exercising four times each week for at least 40 minutes per session.

Please note, that's 40 minutes and four times each week. For many years three times each week for 30 minutes each session was all the rage. But today, researchers and avid exercisers know that there is something magical about those extra ten minutes and about that extra day. Something changes at that level. Try it and you will see that by exercising four days or more each week and at least 40 minutes each session your body will develop a desire to exercise. Your body will actually begin to not just need it, but crave it.

Imagine that! Your body-craving exercise! Wouldn't that be something? Another thing to consider is that obese people's bodies respond more favorably to exercise than thin people. That means that when we exercise, we get more bang for our buck. A bonus!

Well, I am sure that knowing these great things, you are ready right now to go out and exercise, aren't you? Okay, maybe not right now, but remember, you should start slowly and gradually increase the number of minutes that you exercise in your target heart rate. And of course, always check with your physician before starting any sort of exercise program.

EXERCISE FOR WHAT AILS YOU

Through the years we have learned much about the need for and the benefits of exercise. Among others, exercise offers the following benefits:

- Stimulates blood flow

- Stimulates tissue growth in muscle and bone

- Relieves fatigue

- Helps prevent and fight disease

We know that exercise has a great effect on weight loss and makes a significant contribution to our ability to maintain our desired weight. I was quite surprised to learn, however, of the many other health benefits of exercise. I think you, too, will enjoy this research. Exercise has proven to give patients an extra edge when it comes to avoiding or minimizing diseases. Consider the following points from a lecture given at Harvard Medical School by Dr. Herald Elrick:

> *Heart disease.* Exercise helps reverse established disease and helps control the risk factors for heart disease (high blood pressure, high cholesterol, obesity). Exercise also lowers triglycerides and raises high-density lipoproteins (HDL).

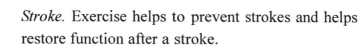

Stroke. Exercise helps to prevent strokes and helps restore function after a stroke.

High blood pressure. Exercise is a non-drug therapy for treating mild-to-moderate high blood pressure, and it helps patients who are on drug therapy for severe high blood pressure.

Diabetes. Exercise can prevent or delay the serious vascular complications of diabetes. Regular exercise can reduce the need for insulin.

Arthritis. Exercise improves endurance, strengthens muscles, and increases joint flexibility and range of motion.

Osteoporosis. Exercise can prevent and reverse bone loss, which can stave off the disabling effects of fractures and bone degeneration.

Depression. Exercise reduces depression and anxiety, increases feelings of well-being, improves the ability to handle stress and improves self-image.

Cancer. Exercise reduces the risk of colon and breast cancer.

Chronic obstructive pulmonary disease. Exercise is an effective rehabilitation component that provides physiologic and psychological benefits.

THE DYNAMIC DUO

Most professionals encourage a combination of both aerobic and strength training to create a well-balanced and comprehensive exercise regimen. It is important that we understand the differences and the benefits of each type of exercise.

AEROBIC TRAINING

The word aerobic means, "with oxygen." Aerobic strength is getting the oxygen needed to your working muscles and removing the buildup of waste products. It is also referred to as "cardiovascular endurance." Aerobic activities are usually long in duration and low in intensity. Activities like walking, biking, swimming, cross-country skiing are all considered aerobic. During these activities you should be able to talk normally. If you find yourself gasping for air, it is likely that you are working anaerobically. Anaerobic activities are short in duration and high in intensity. Racquetball, downhill skiing, weight lifting, sprinting, football, and soccer are usually anaerobic.

Benefits of aerobic exercise:

- Conditions the heart and lungs.

- Controls body fat stores.

- Increases energy and resistance to fatigue.

- Decreases tension and aids in sleeping.

- Psychological benefits include: improved mood, reduced depression and anxiety.

STRENGTH TRAINING

Strength training also has many short-term and long-term benefits. Some of the primary benefits are that it improves endurance and increases lean muscle mass and muscle strength. It also improves balance, flexibility, mobility and stability. Other benefits include the following:

- Increases and restores bone density.

- Increases the body's metabolic rate, which aids the body in burning more calories.

- Improving skill and performance in sports programs.

- Helping appearance, because people look and feel better and because stronger muscles and joints can have a dramatic affect on posture.

I am pleased to be able to introduce you to a WLS exerciser whom I have admired for many years. She is one who smartly exchanged her love for food for a love for exercise. She is a healthy and fit long term loser and spends her life motivating and inspiring others to make exercise an integral part of their day.

TAMMY BARTZ, CPT

My battle with weight began at the early age of 9. By age 10, I weighed 125 lbs. As is the case with so many people, food was a comfort and coping tool for me. The wrong foods were readily available and I always seemed to have

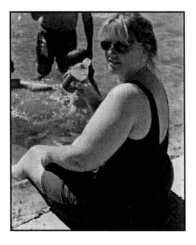

an overwhelming urge to eat until it was all gone. One cookie led to one row, then two, and then the bag.

My first diet was at the age of 11. During my sophomore year of high school I discovered Dexatrim, diet Coke, and starvation. I lost about 30 lbs only to regain it once again. From there it was every diet I could get my hands on. Then came along Phen-Fen, and I successfully lost but soon regained double the pounds.

In 1997, I reached my all time high of 269 lbs. At 5'5" that was more than my knees, back and self-esteem could handle.

My mother, also struggled with her weight and together we fought what seemed like an endless, losing battle. In 1999 my mother scheduled an appointment with a Salt Lake City surgeon to discuss having gastric bypass. I went with her to find all the faults and show her that it was too drastic and there would surely be another way; you know, more diet and exercise. "Ha!" After meeting with her surgeon, and reading him the riot act, he, unknowingly convinced me to be open to the idea that this could be my solution, too. After doing further research, attending BSCI's "Surgical Solutions" presentation and several support groups, I had the confidence to move forward. I admit that I was scared to death but knew this would be the tool I needed to help control my life long battle with weight.

I successfully reached my goal before my one-year check-up. I lost a whole person. This has been great for my family, too because they are much more aware of their food and exercise habits. I can fit comfortably in a movie theatre seat, my rear doesn't hang over the chair, and I can get in and out of bathroom stall with ease. My knees and low back rarely bother me anymore. I can tie my shoes without passing out from lack of oxygen.

Now, at 7 years post op and weighing 120 pounds, it's a whole new world for me. I exercise daily. Imagine that; I exercise every day! I have become an avid exerciser. It has become part of my lifestyle and includes a variety of strength and aerobic exercises. This has resulted in the "firm success" I have enjoyed. One year after my surgery I ran a 5k in under 30 minutes! It was such a thrill to be able to do that! I received my certification as a personal trainer in 2002. My book, Strength-n-Sculpt (BSCI 2005), was written to help bariatric patients customize a routine that works for them. Finding "fitness that fits" is the key to making exercise a part of your life.

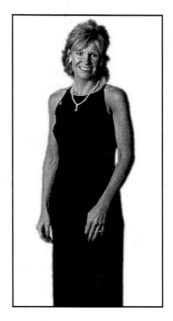

Today, I continue to be thrilled with the comments of old friends and associates who ask, "Your voice sounds so familiar but who are you?" Or, "Did you do something to your hair?"

TAKE THE
SUCCESS HABITS™ CHALLENGE!

Aerobic and Strength Exercise

1. Add a new exercise to your routine. If you are doing mostly aerobic exercises add some strength training. If you are doing primarily strength training, add an aerobic workout to your routine.

2. Push yourself a little. Add 1 mile or an extra 10 minutes to your workout.

Success Habits™ Principle 5
Regular Exercise

DAILY CHECK-UP QUESTIONS

✔

I exercised today.   Yes ☐ No ☐

I exercised within my target
heart rate zone today.   Yes ☐ No ☐

I made an effort to be more
"active" today.   Yes ☐ No ☐

Success Habits™ Principle 6

Vitamins and Supplements

*"I take good quality vitamins each day
to ensure my good health."*

Critics of weight-loss surgery contend that in the long run, vitamin deficiencies run rampant among weight-loss surgery patients. There were some significant deficiencies resulting from early bariatric procedures but much has been learned about absorption issues in patients, as well as the need for supplementation. As weight-loss surgery patients, we must take personal accountability for our health and long-term well-being by complying with our doctors' recommendations to supplement our diets with necessary vitamins and nutrients. All patients are encouraged to take a high quality multi-vitamin as well as a calcium supplement each day. As needed, others are required to take supplemental iron and/or B12.

Most bariatric surgeons recommend that weight-loss surgery patients have their blood work done at least annually to ensure that their bodies are receiving and absorbing the proper vitamins and nutrients for life-long good health.

In this chapter we will discuss the importance of nutritional supplements in weight-loss surgery patients, learn about calcium, iron, B12, issues related to bariatric patients and review common recommendations for annual blood tests and screenings.

I have always known that taking vitamins should be a routine part of my day. I have been at least somewhat compliant, but for a weight-loss surgery patient, "somewhat" is not enough. Early on I made the commitment to have my blood work done each year in the month of my bariatri surgery anniversary. For the first few years, my tests came back within normal ranges and I, of course, was pleased, thinking that I had a handle on my health. With that attitude, I became lax in taking my vitamins. I missed an annual checkup or two and before I knew it several years had gone by without having my blood work done.

It is important to me that I "walk my talk," that I live the principles I teach, that I comply with all of the Success Habits™ principles myself. But months and years passed. I began to hear comments like, "You look tired," and "Are you feeling OK?" I have been known to be a work-aholic, so I dismissed their comments and ignored how run down I was feeling. It seemed that each day I would have this same conversation with myself, "I know, I should have my blood work done. I know I should take my vitamins. But life... well, finally there were no more excuses!

And so, I had my blood work done and the results

kicked me in the butt! My B-12 level was dangerously low, so I started taking shots once each week. At first, Ingrid, my nurse, was giving them to me. Then, she taught my daughter Miranda how to do it. (Not too much fun for a teenager to give her mom a B-12 shot in the butt!)

So, then, my husband, who is scared of needles, agreed to try it once. As he did, I could see his reflection in our bathroom mirror and he was getting a run at it! "Wait!!!! No thank you, I will do it myself," I said. After all, how hard could it be. My fanny is a lot smaller than it used to be and easier to reach and it was just a little shot anyway. So, bravely, I gave myself a little stick, pressed the syringe and squeezed. I was quite proud of myself, for about a nano-second, until I realized that the B-12 was running down the back of my leg. I had not even broken the skin! What a wimp. Anyway, I do much better now. I have given myself a B-12 shot each week for about 6 months now and can real-ly tell a difference in my energy level.

Having my blood tests results prompted me to examine my understanding of and compliance with this important success habit principle. As you read this chapter, my hope is that you will take responsibility for your own health by hav-ing your blood work done, and then keep it in check by committing to take high quality vitamins and supplements.

It has been my good fortune and now yours to learn from the work of Dr. Jacqueline Jacques. Dr. Jacques is an accomplished and sought-after professional in the field of vitamins, supplements and nutrient absorption. She is the principal reseacher for Bariatric Advantage (see Appendix A, Helpful People, Products, and Programs) and is responsible for developing the formulary for their vitamins, which have been created to meet the specific needs of weight-loss surgery patients. With her permission, I have included one of her informative articles here. It is entitled "The Importance of Nutritional Supplements in Weight-Loss Surgery":

You may have noticed in the news recently that the American Medical Association now recommends that all Americans would likely benefit from taking a daily multivitamin and mineral supplement[1]. Why? Because few if any of us are able to meet the daily requirements of the nutrients we need through the foods we eat. In addition to this, some disease conditions (such as diabetes) can predispose a person to specific nutritional deficiencies, and medications may deplete or inhibit the absorption of others.

This issue becomes more complicated in patients who have had weight-loss surgery.[2] To get nutrients (from either food or supplements) to our cells, they first must pass through the digestive system. Different nutrients are broken down and absorbed in different parts of the digestive system, so when the system is surgically altered, challenges arise. Also, most vitamins and minerals can be found in a variety of chemical forms, and the chemical form may have a great effect on how well the nutrient is digested and used by the body.

In the most common form of weight-loss surgery, the Roux-en-Y gastric bypass, the stomach is reduced to a small pouch and much of the duodenum is bypassed. It is important that weight-loss surgery patients understand how these changes affect their vitamin and mineral absorption.

• The smaller size of the stomach, along with pre-scribed diets, means fewer calories are consumed; and this means fewer nutrients are eaten.

• There is less contact with stomach acid, and some nutrients require acid for processing.

• There is less contact, and perhaps less production of a substance called Intrinsic Factor, which is needed for vitamin B12 absorption.

• Many important nutrients were absorbed primari-ly in the duodenum, so they may also become defi-cient when the duodenum has been bypassed.

Because the quality of a supplement and the forms of the specific nutrients can have a great impact on the body's ability to absorb and utilize them, it is important to choose a product that meets the highest standards. Things to look for in a high quality supplement are:

> • *Use of nutrients that are USP (made according to the United States Pharmacopoeia)*

> • *Use of nutrients that are pharmaceutical grade. Pharmaceutical grade nutrients have very small, uniform particle sizes and are easier to absorb.*

> • *Products manufactured in a pharmaceutically licensed facility-which means that they must use the same strict standards that apply to drug manufacturers.*

> • *Products tested by FDA approved methods for their ability to dissolve and disintegrate; this means they will break down in your digestive system.[3]*

Also look for forms of nutrients such as citrates and gluconates that are easy on the digestive system. This is especially important for minerals like iron that can cause digestive upset and constipation if a gentle form is not used. Natural forms of nutrients may also be more bioavailable, and are thus pre-ferred to synthetic forms. Since the needs of weight-loss surgery patients are much more specialized than those of the average person, it may be best to choose a product that has been designed with your surgery in mind.

For patients who have undergone weight-loss surgery it may be necessary to take some nutrients in higher doses (such as calcium), or in different forms (such as B12, which may be best delivered under the tongue). Your doctor will follow your nutritional status periodically through lab tests and may make recommendations that are specific to your needs.[4]

Nutritional supplements are generally best absorbed if taken with a meal. Your body likes you to spread your food out into several small meals daily; you will get the most out of your vitamins if you do the same. The most important thing to remember about your vitamins is that they won't work and they can't help you if you don't take them. It may be helpful to carry them with you in a pillbox and keep another at home and yet another at work so that you can't forget. Taking your supplements daily is an important part of supporting your health goals. Complying with this Success Habit as well as the other five can help you to achieve greater, life-long well-being.

– Jacqueline Jacques, ND Medical/Nutritional Advisor, Bariatric Advantage

THE FACTS ABOUT CALCIUM

Calcium is needed for the heart, muscles and nerves to function properly and for blood to clot. Inadequate calcium is thought to contribute to the development of osteoporosis. National nutrition surveys have shown that many women and young girls consume less than half the recommended daily allowance (RDA) of calcium.

Vegetables such as broccoli and carrots, fish like shrimp and salmon, and low-fat and non-fat dairy products are all good sources of calcium.

For weight-loss surgery patients, the recommended daily allowance of calcium is 1200 mg. per day. More than 2,000 mg. of calcium per day is not recommended as it may increase the likelihood of developing kidney stones in people who are prone to them.

Calcium Citrate is the best choice and is best absorbed on an empty stomach.

Calcium is best absorbed if taken in amounts of 500 mg. or less several times a day.

Calcium has always been something that has been difficult for me to take as often throughout the day as I should. I was thrilled when I heard about the new "Viactiv" Calcium Supplements that came out a while back. They are like caramels, yum, but much to my dismay, are made of calci-

TAKE THE
SUCCESS HABITS™ CHALLENGE!

Calcium

1. Make arrangements to have a Bone Density Test. For more information call your healthcare provider.

2. Identify the type of calcium you are currently taking. If you are taking calcium carbonate, switch to the more absorbable form, or a "citrate" based calcium.

um carbonate, not calcium citrate. Oh well, I thought. Someday someone will make a calcium supplement that makes sense. Well, that day has finally arrived. They are calcium citrate in the form of a mint lozenge! I am thrilled to recommend yet another one of Bariatric Advantage's products (see Helpful Products and Programs in the Appendix for contact information).

THE IMPORTANCE OF VITAMIN B12

Vitamin B12, also called cobalamin, is important to good health. Its function is to help maintain healthy nerve cells and red blood cells. B12 is also needed to make DNA. Supplemental B12, the acid in the stomach that releases B12 from protein during digestion, is especially important for most weight-loss surgery patients. Once released, B12 combines with a substance called intrinsic factor before it is absorbed into the bloodstream. The lower portion of the stomach produces both acid and intrinsic factor. After weight-loss surgery, the lower part of the stomach aids somewhat in this process, but not at its former capacity.

B12 deficiency may occur as a result of an inability to break down and absorb B12 from food. It can also occur in individuals with dietary patterns that exclude animal or for-tified foods such as vegetarian or vegan diets. B12 defi-ciency can lead to neurological changes such as numbness and tingling in the hands and feet. Additional symptoms of B12 deficiency are difficulty in maintaining balance, depression, confusion, poor memory, and soreness of the mouth or tongue. Some of these symptoms can also result from a variety of medical conditions other than vitamin B12 deficiency. It is important to have a physician evaluate these symptoms so that appropriate medical care can be given.

The most common characteristic signs of B12 deficiency include fatigue, weakness, nausea, constipation, flatulence (gas), loss of appetite, and weight loss.

There are a number of sources for B12. First, vitamin B12 is naturally found in animal foods including fish, milk and milk products, eggs, meat, and poultry. Fortified breakfast cereals are also an excellent source of vitamin B12. In addition to getting B12 from food, it is available in pill form, liquid, spray, sublingually, or as a shot. If B12 levels are low, weekly B12 shots will often be recommended. For normal levels, the best therapy is usually sublingual ingestion.

I have often wondered and been asked if one can get too much B12. The Institute of Medicine states:

"No adverse effects have been associated with excess vitamin B12 intake from food and supplements in healthy individuals."

So, how do you know if you are maintaining proper levels of B12? Once again, it is recommended that weight-loss surgery patients have their B12 levels checked at least once

TAKE THE
SUCCESS HABITS™ CHALLENGE!

Vitamin B-12

1. Make arrangements to have a blood test specifically for B12 Levels. A serum B12 test is often used but for early detection a test of homocysteine levels is recommended.

2. If a B12 supplement is needed, try either a sublingual or a B12 injection.

each year and have the results sent to their bariatric surgeon's office for evaluation. Many simply order serum B12 levels, but according to Dr. Jacques, early detection is vitally important, so she recommends that homocysteine levels be checked more frequently, than once per year.

ANNUAL CHECKUP AND BLOOD WORK

Bariatric professionals encourage all weight-loss surgery patients to have their blood work done each year to ensure that their bodies are getting and absorbing the many vitamins and minerals necessary for good health. The following tests are recommended annually:

1. *Comprehensive metabolic panel.* The Comprehensive Metabolic Panel (CMP) is a group of 14 tests that provides important information about the current status of your kidneys, liver, and electrolyte and acid-base balance as well as of your blood sugar and blood proteins.

2. *Lipid profile.* The lipid profile is a group of tests that are often ordered together to determine risk of coronary heart disease. These tests that have been shown to be good indicators of whether someone is likely to have a heart attack or stroke caused by blockage of blood vessels or "hardening of the arteries". The lipid profile includes total cholesterol, HDL-cholesterol (often called good cholesterol),

LDL-cholesterol (often called bad cholesterol), and triglycerides.

3. *Complete blood count.* One of the most important blood tests is called a complete blood count (CBC). While there are many different types of cells in your blood, they can all be grouped into one of three categories: red blood cells, white blood cells, and platelets. Knowing how many of these cells you have in a blood sample provides a lot of valuable information about the condition of your health.

4. *B12 level.* Vitamin B12 testing usually consists of two tests. The first is a serum B12 blood test to measure the amount of B12 in the blood. The second is a test to rule out any folic acid deficiency, which can mimic the symptoms of B12 deficiency.

TAKE THE
SUCCESS HABITS™ CHALLENGE!

Annual Blood Work

1. Make arrangements to have your annual blood work done per your bariatric surgeon's guidelines.

2. Request a copy for yourself and begin a file for you to keep at home. Compare to other years if available. Report any and all items of concern to your physician or surgeon.

3. Learn more about reading your blood test results.

VITAMINS IN ALL THEIR VARIETIES

Weight-loss surgery patients are encouraged to take a high quality vitamin & supplements each day. Multi-vitamins are available in a variety of forms and one should pay close attention to the content, quality and especially the absorbability. Different forms of vitamins have different features, costs and absorption levels. Vitamins are available in a variety of forms, a few of which are listed below.

• Chewable - New weight-loss surgery patients often begin with easy-to-swallow chewables. Even though these vitamins are often referred to as children's vitamins, it is important to take the adult dosage as recommended.

• Tablet - Most name-brand vitamins come in tablet form. Be aware, however, that generic tablets may have an outer shell that could make absorption difficult.

• Capsule - Capsules can be swallowed whole, or opened and the contents mixed into soft foods such as yogurt or cottage cheese.

• Liquid – Weight-loss surgery patients may prefer to use a liquid form of vitamin rather than one of the pill varieties. Many name-brand vitamins are now available in liquid form.

Recommendations vary from procedure to procedure and doctor to doctor and unfortunately at this point there are no uniform protocols. However, here are common recommendations for a variety of bariatric surgical procedures:

LapBand®
Multi Vitamin alone
Multi Vitamin, Calcium, & B-12

Gastric Bypass
Chewable Multi Vitamin
Sublingual B-12
Calcium
Sometimes Iron

Duodenal Switch
Multi Vitamin with added fat-soluble vitamins (A,D,E, and K)
Calcium (usually a high dose 1500 - 2500 mg)
Sometimes Iron & B-12
Sometimes EFAs

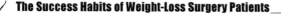
• Spray – For many years, athletes have utilized this unique method of taking vitamins. Spray vitamins are thought to increase the speed and the amount of absorption and are a good choice for weight-loss surgery patients.

• Sub-lingual – B12 is one vitamin known to be well absorbed sublingually, or under the tongue. Usually sublingual supplements and vitamins are made with a pleasing taste and are made to absorb slowly.

In addition to vitamin absorbability it is important to understand that our bodies need supplementation more than once a day. The best way to be sure you are getting the best absorption of all your vitamins each day is to develop the habit of taking vitamins with each meal - three times each day. Carry them with you, so no matter where you are when you eat out you always have your vitamins. Experience tells us that vitamins which have been specifically formulated for weight-loss surgery patients are both necessary and superior to generic vitamins that can be purchased over the counter.

TAKE THE
SUCCESS HABITS™ CHALLENGE!

Vitamins

1. If your bariatric surgeon has not recommended any particular vitamin, do some investigating and comparison shopping yourself. There are few vitamins especially formulated for weight-loss patients.

2. Take the time to distribute your vitamins in several different places to remind you to take them several times each day. Keep a supply in your purse, car, desk, kitchen, and bathroom.

3. It is important to understand that our bodies need supplementation more than once a day. I have made a habit of taking vitamins with each meal–three times each day. I carry them with me, so no matter where I am, I always have my vitamins.

4. It has been my experience that the vitamins which have been specifically formulated for weight-loss surgery patients are far superior to anything that can be purchased over the counter (see Appendix A, Helpful People, Programs, and Products).

Success Habits™ Principle 6
Vitamins and Suplements

DAILY CHECK-UP QUESTIONS

My blood work has been done
within the past 12 months.   Yes ☐   No ☐

I took a high quality multivitamin
today.   Yes ☐   No ☐

I took my calcium, iron and B12, if
prescribed.   Yes ☐   No ☐

Back On Track

Well, it happens. We never thought it could, we promised ourselves we wouldn't let it, but the fact remains, we've re-gained weight. For some, just a few innocent pounds, but for others many unwanted pounds. Pounds they thought they would never see again. When weight gain occurs, accepting responsibility for screwing up the best thing that ever happened to you is next to impossible. Notice I said, "next" to impossible.

THE END OF INVINCIBLE

Success! Finally. A lifetime of struggling, losing, gaining, gaining, losing were finally over. I had found the answer: weight-loss surgery. And what a needed and most welcome solution it was. The first two years following my surgery were unbelievable. Looking back it seemed that the weight just fell off! And then I was normal, thin and healthy. I wore a size 6! And apparently I am a tiny, petite, small-framed person. Who knew?

I had succeeded, finally! I was a winner and I was in control. It seemed that now I had a handle on things, I could relax a bit. I had worked so hard, now it was time to enjoy the rewards. It seemed I could eat just about anything. Once in a while, I would have a little cookie here, a little piece of candy there without gaining, then a bite of cake or pie. I could slack off a bit on my exercise and the scales remained the same. "This is great," I thought, "finally, some reprieve from all the worry, all the disappointments. I am just like a normal person now. Just like those who I have seen eat whatever they want, never exercise and always remain thin and healthy."

And then it happened. I started to regain. Three pounds, then five, then seven. The horror that I felt helped me to recognize that I had reached a very important milestone. A milestone that I have termed "The End of Invincible."(See Appendix D for my 10 year weight loss progress chart.)

Obesity is a disease much like alcoholism; there is no "cure." Rather, there are habits one can develop to treat the disease through the remainder of life. I recognize now more than ever that I am not normal; my body is different than that of a thin person. It metabolizes food differently; it requires constant monitoring of the calories in/calories out balance to maintain a healthy weight. While I had won the battle, the war was still going on and whenever I turned my back on it, I would be struck with another pound or two. I came to recognize that I have to be constantly on guard, constantly in control, forever monitoring, and tirelessly committed to the Success Habits™ principles.

Each success habit is important in its own right, but it is the constant adherence to ALL of them that fosters life-long change.

One thing I know for sure is that weight-loss surgery patients are some of the strongest, most resilient, committed, never-say-never people I have ever met.

We are well acquainted with failure. We know what it takes to pick ourselves up, dust ourselves off and do whatever it takes to meet our goals. But as experienced as we are with winning and losing, admitting and taking responsibility for our failures is never easy, but we must learn to become successful failures.

I don't like whipped cream. Never have, never will. I don't like the taste or the texture. But bless their hearts, the staff arranged a special diet dessert for the company Christmas party: a frothy whipped cream pie made with diet cool whip, yogurt and sugarless Jello. Dinner was great, and it was so thoughtful of them to give those of us who are patients an alternative to the ever-delicious Mudd Pie. I declined both dessert options and enjoyed the fresh strawberries instead. Well, that was until it was time to go home.

There was one slice of diet pie left, which I slyly took and placed on my tray. I hid it securely beneath a napkin; heaven forbid that one of the surgeons see me smuggling a piece of diet pie out of the room! As we drove down the mountain from this lovely resort cabin, I lifted the napkin off of the whipped cream pie and began to eat it with my fingers. Did I mention that I hate whipped cream? Nevertheless, I ate it…with my fingers. I offered a handful to my husband who declined as he gave me a strange look that I could only see by the dashboard lights. What a sticky mess. I don't know what got into me, but I do know that I ate the whole thing! With my fingers, in the dark.

We stopped on the way home to do a little shopping at an outlet store. As I got out of the truck, I saw the first glimpse of myself in the parking lot lights. I was wearing a black jump suit, full-length black coat, black boots, and scarf. And I had pink whipped cream all over myself. In an attempt to cover up my misdeeds, I flipped the lapel of my coat over to reveal the clean underside; but to no avail. The look on the clerk's face when I entered her store told me it was apparent to her that I was quite a partier! I have never been so embarrassed in all my life. I felt like such a slob, such a pig, such an undisciplined failure. It seemed that, for some unexplainable reason, I could not control my behavior. The whipped cream pie had beaten me. Why? I have analyzed and analyzed. I have wondered and questioned. I have beaten myself up over and over again. I don't know exactly why this happened, but I can tell you that I will never, never eat anything with whipped cream again! Ever!

I share this story with you becuause I belive you undoubtedly have your own food obsession stories, hang-ups and temptations. You have your own whipped cream pie story. May I encourage you to recognize it, analyze it and learn from your experience to recognize your mistakes, take responsibility for them, own them, learn from them and do whatever it takes to become a "successful failure".

A number of years ago I was getting ready for work, listening to the radio and there was a report on about the NASA space shuttle that was getting ready to lift off. All of a sudden, something went wrong and they canceled it all. On the radio they were calling it a "successful failure." I thought, "A successful failure, isn't that interesting?" It was an oxymoron. So I went downstairs to turn on the television to see what had happened. The space shuttle was ready to go, all the money had been spent to launch it, the astronauts were on board, everything was a go. The countdown came: five…four…three, … at three minutes to lift off, the computer sensed there was something wrong and shut everything down. It didn't launch. That is why they called it a successful failure. Do you remember the space shuttle Challenger? Do you remember there were lives lost? That was a failure. A real failure. I believe that, in our lives, anything that we do that is a failure can be, and should be viewed as, a successful failure. Many of the things that happen in our lives are so etched on our hearts and in our minds with such great emotion and hurt and pain, that we don't even want to think about them, let alone learn from them. It is important that you take some time for introspection, to look at your life, at some of the things that you have been through. Identify how you can learn from those experiences to become a successful failure.

Perhaps you have read the little children's book, *The Velveteen Rabbit*. Let me recap part of it for you. In the nursery there were all kinds of toys: new ones, old ones, fluffy ones and wind up toys. The oldest toy in the nursery was the old Skin Horse. And the newest toy in the nursery was the Velveteen Rabbit. The Velveteen Rabbit and the old Skin Horse were having a conversation:

> *"What is real?" asked the Rabbit one day. "Does is mean having things that buzz inside of you and a stick out handle?"*

> *"Real isn't how you are made. It's a thing that happens to you. When a child loves you for a long, long time, not just to play with, but REALLY loves you. Then you become real."*

> *"Does it hurt?" asked the Rabbit.*

"Sometimes," said the Skin Horse for he was always truthful. "When you are Real you don't mind being hurt."

"Does it happen all at once, like being wound up," he asked, "or bit by bit?"

"It doesn't happen all at once," said the Skin Horse. "You become. It takes a long time. That's why it doesn't often happen to people who break easily, or have sharp edges, or who have to be carefully kept. Generally, by the time you are Real most of your hair has been loved off, and your eyes drop out, and you get loose in the joints and very shabby. But these things don't matter at all, because once you are Real you can't be ugly, except to people who don't understand." (*The Velveteen Rabbit* by Margery Williams)

Now I ask, do you feel real? Do you have enough in your life to feel like a real person? We all have failures, disappointments, difficulties, and challenges.

THE OLD WOMAN

Many years ago I was speaking at a women's conference at a restaurant in downtown Salt Lake City. I was in charge of the meeting; I was the motivator. I was on top of it all;

ready to go and everything was going well. The sales people and staff were positive and it was a beautiful spring day. I had on a turquoise suit (size 24, mind you), but nevertheless, I was all that and a bag of chips, and I was ready to go to my meeting.

As I was walking down the street early that morning. I saw coming toward me, an old woman. She was old, old, old, very tall and lanky, her hair was all messy, and she was kind of hunched over. She wasn't carrying a bag or a briefcase or a purse or a suitcase or even a garbage sack. She wasn't carrying anything at all. She was just scary looking, like the old Maleficent, or one of the other childhood witches we were frightened of. And I thought, "Ohhh, I am certainly glad I'm not her." And as we got a little bit closer, I could see that her eyes were all black and blue inside, blood shot, and her teeth were all rotted out. And she had long, long, pointy, dirty, filthy, awful fingernails. And I just got a terrible awful feeling, and was thinking, "Ohhh, I am so glad that I am not her."

And as we got closer on the sidewalk, and as our eyes met, she said to me, "My you're fat and ugly!" I did not know what to say. I didn't know what to think. You don't know whether to laugh or cry for me, do you? Well, two steps later I was at my meeting and I had to kind of slap myself on the cheek a little bit because it was show time. I had to go and do and be what I needed to be.

This instance was only one of the little jabs, the little hurts, the little stabs, the little things that hurt me because of my weight and where I was in my life. I learned from those kinds of experiences, the trying and failing, year after year after year. But finally, I made a decision that was right for me, right for my health. And finally, I became a successful failure.

THE RACE

"Quit! Give up! You're beaten!" they shout at me and plead,
"There's just too much against you now, this time you can't succeed."
And as I start to hang my head in front of failure's face,
My downward fall is broken by the memory of a race.
And hope refills my weakened will as I recall that scene,
For just the thought of that short race rejuvenates my being.
A children's race, young boys, young men, how I remember well,
Excitement, sure! But also fear, it wasn't hard to tell.
They all lined up so full of hope each thought to win that race,
Or tie for first, or if not that, at least take second place.
And fathers watched from off the side, each cheering for his son,
And each boy hoped to show his dad that he would be the one.
The whistle blew and off they went, young hearts and hopes afire,
To win and be the hero there was each young boy's desire.
And one boy in particular whose dad was in the crowd,
Was running in the lead and thought, "My dad will be so proud!"
But as they speeded down the field, across a shallow dip,

The little boy who thought to win, lost his step and slipped.

Trying hard to catch himself, his hands flew out to brace,

And mid the laughter of the crowd, he fell flat on his face.

So down he fell and with him hope; he couldn't win it now.

Embarrassed, sad, he only wished to disappear somehow.

But as he fell his dad stood up and showed his anxious face,

Which to the boy so clearly said, "Get up and win that race."

He quickly rose, no damage done, behind a bit, that's all,

And ran with all his mind and might to make up for his fall.

So anxious to restore himself, to catch up and to win,

His mind went faster than his legs, he slipped and fell again!

He wished then he had quit before with only one disgrace.

"I'm hopeless as a runner now; I shouldn't try to race."

But in the laughing crowd he searched and found his father's face;

That steady look which said again, "Get up and win that race!"

So up he jumped to try again, ten yards behind the last,

"If I'm to gain those yards," he thought, I've got to move real fast."

Exerting everything he had he regained eight or ten,

But trying hard to catch the lead he slipped and fell again!

Defeat! He lay there silently. A tear dropped from his eye.

"There's no sense running anymore. Three strikes, I'm out! Why try?"

The will to rise had disappeared, all hope had fled away,

So far behind, so error prone, a loser all the way.

"I've lost, so what's the use," he thought, "I'll live with my disgrace."

But then he thought about his dad, who soon he'd have to face.

"Get up," an echo sounded low. "Get up and take your place,

You were not meant for failure here, Get up and win that race."

With borrowed will "Get up," it said, "You haven't lost at all,

For winning is no more than this: to rise each time you fall."

So up he rose to run once more, and with a new commit,

He resolved that win or lose, at least he wouldn't quit.

So far behind the others now, the most he'd ever been,

Still he gave it all he had, and ran as though to win.

Three times he'd fallen, stumbling, three times he rose again,

Too far behind to hope to win, he still ran to the end.

They cheered the winning runner, as he crossed the line first place.

Head high, and proud, and happy; no failing, no disgrace.

But when the fallen youngster, crossed the line last place,

The crowd gave him the greater cheer, for finishing the race.

And even though he came in last, with head bowed low, unproud,

You would have thought he'd won the race, to listen to the crowd.

And to his dad he sadly said, "I didn't do so well."

"To me, you won," his father said, "You rose each time you fell."

And now when things seem dark and hard and difficult to face,

The memory of that little boy helps me in my own race.

For all of life is like that race, with ups and downs and all,

And all you have to do to win is rise each time you fall

"Quit!" "Give up!" "You're beaten!" they still shout in my face,

But another voice within me says, "GET UP AND WIN THAT RACE!

    – Anonymous

I wish I knew who wrote this inspirational poem, but the writer is anonymous. Isn't it a wonderful story? For winning is not more than this, but to rise each time you fall."

Never see failure as failure, but only as a chance to change your course. If you find yourself at an undesirable weight be willing to take some risks, embrace a challenge. Always keep in mind that if you are not falling, if you are not failing, if you are not encountering stumbling blocks, difficulties and challenges in your life, you are probably not going anywhere either. So I encourage you to learn to become a successful failure. Pick yourself up, dust yourself off and do whatever it takes.

"So, just what does it take to get back on track?" You may be wondering. Well here is what I have learned.

Through the years I've noticed that as patients regain extra pounds they swore they would never see again, they are so devastated with feelings of guilt, hopelessness and regret that they stop attending support groups and refuse to see their bariatric surgeons. Some are so distraught that they will not even acknowledge they have had weight-loss surgery at all. I have seen many, through the years, desperately needing help and not knowing where to turn. Some have rejoined old weight loss programs such as Weight Watchers International, Inc.® or Jenny Craig; Inc.®, others have started the Atkins Diet™ again. Others even turn to prescriptions for weight-loss pills and powders.

Recognizing the need for a program for these faltering patients, I began a monthly "Back On Track" class in 1998. Understanding the unique physiology and specific needs of bariatric patients, I customized this program to meet those needs. Patients who have regained weight, often uncomfortable in support groups, find this class to be welcoming, helpful and motivating.

This Back on Track program has met with great success. Patients recognize that their bodies are different and that the "tool" they have been given through bariatric surgery is still a tool that will serve them well, as long as they use it properly. Using our Success Habits™ principles as the foundation, we help patients understand, incorporate and internalize these winning principles.

BSCI's Back On Track Programs today includes tele-seminars, online learning modules, back on track forums and new Back On Track Resource Booklet program. More details are available at www.bariatricsupportcenter.com.

If you have regained weight, you can still use the Success Habits™ principles to lose the weight and then maintain your weight loss.

FEARING SUCCESS

Television brings us entertainment, but once in a while, it brings us a great message. Such was the case with an episode of a popular show, Chicago Hope, that I saw several years ago. The story was told of a man who was admitted into the emergency room with stomach pains. He had concocted a special dietary drink to help him lose weight. He had lost weight rapidly but did it in such an unhealthy way he caused some damage to his body in the process. The emergency room team evaluated him and decided the immediate course of action would be to pump the harmful substance out of his stomach. After the urgent care, the ER doctor sat down beside the young man and explained that he had put himself at great risk with this homemade remedy. He acknowledged that his excessive weight was also unhealthy and suggested that the patient see a colleague of his that had great success with weight-loss surgery for weight control. "WOW," I thought. Prime time TV was recognizing the surgical treatment, at least as an option.

I waited patiently for the young man's response to the doctor's suggestion. "That would never work for me," he said, "anyway, I would never do something that drastic to my body." "Oh, the irony," I thought. And then the doctor counseled him, suggesting that he recognize that he was not afraid that the surgery would fail, he suspected that the young man was afraid that the surgery would succeed.

The show continued with another story line, but at the end of the program, the young man returned to the hospital and asked to meet with the ER doctor that had treated him several weeks earlier. Looking much better and on the road to recovery from the former incident, he thanked the doctor for his treatment and quietly confessed, "I have been thinking, doctor. I realized that you're right about that surgery option. I am not afraid that the surgery will fail; I am afraid the surgery will succeed. You see I have failed at almost everything in my life. And as I have, I have blamed all my failures on my weight. I can't hold a job because I am too fat. I don't go out for sports, because I am a couch potato. I am a slob because I can't find clothes that fit me. I don't date because I am not attractive. My entire life I have blamed everything on my weight. And if weight-loss surgery were to succeed, what would I blame my shortcomings on?"

What a profound message. So often we see patients who, when they get close to their goal weight, sabotage their own success. They are truly afraid to succeed. Success can be quite an adjustment. Following significant weight loss, patients feel different and look different, and people treat them differently; a scary place to be for some. If thoughts of your new self frighten you, if you feel that you might be afraid of success, then you may want to analyze your motives for losing weight. Are you doing this for someone else? Are you concerned that others in your life will have a hard time adjusting? There may be many things contributing to your fears.

In her study, *Intimate Saboteurs*, Dr. Gaye Andrews presented several case studies about successful weight-loss patients who, having reached their goal weight, found great discord in other areas of their life and subsequently chose to have the procedure reversed.

Emotional and relationship issues are certainly something that many must face and deal with. One thing to keep in mind is that bariatric surgery is surgery on your body, not your brain. Some patients find that psychological counseling is helpful as they adjust to the changes in their bodies. Others find support at classes or support group meetings or online.

A Six Year Post-Op Complication

I had a good handle on my eating habits: I was a pretty good exerciser and I drank a lot of water. All seemed well, except for that little pain in my stomach. I woke up to this pain on occasion throughout the six years since my surgery. Usually, once I got up and moved around a bit, the pain would go away. It felt like something was stuck.

Sometimes a little sip of water or a Saltine cracker would do the trick. It was my gallbladder, I was quite sure. But one morning in February 2000, the pain did not go away; rather, it got worse and worse. Assuming it would subside as it had done before, I went about my normal daily routine.

Instead of subsiding, the pain grew steadily worse and by early afternoon, I acknowledged the need for medical attention. The physician and I were convinced that I needed my gallbladder removed, so we proceeded. My husband met me at the emergency room where I was pumped full of drugs, but regardless, the pain continued to worsen. To my good fortune, my bariatric surgeon, Dr. Smith was available to attend to me and removed my gallbladder.

Suspecting, however, that this was not the only problem, he ordered more tests. I began throwing up blood and bile in quantities unheard of for a weight-loss surgery patient. The doctors found a very rare complication, termed 'reverse' intra-susception, wherein a small part of my bowel had telescoped over itself from the bottom to the top, just below the anastamosis. I was taken back into surgery where they removed that section of bowel. It was a strange and rare complication to be sure.

All is well now, but I share this with you to impress upon your mind that as a weight-loss surgery patient you must be ever-aware that you are not invincible! You have undergone a major alteration to your digestive system. You are different. And it is likely that your primary care physician may not be familiar with your new anatomy and how to help you, should you need attention. You must take responsibility for your life-long good health by staying in close contact with your support center and your bariatric surgeon's office through the years.

When Dreams Come True...Then What?

I was an adorable baby, all rolly-poly. I was a darling little girl, you know, kind of chubby. I was a pretty teen, just sort of pleasingly plump. I became a lovely young woman, but kind of heavy set. Then one day someone pointed me out by saying, "That fat woman." All of my life I have been who I am, plus some sort of explanation. I became myself comma, my weight.

Growing up, each of us may have been labeled as this sort or that sort. Throughout our lives as obese people, we have created many new labels for ourselves to compensate or to distract people or to re-focus their attention on something other than our appearance. We became, "The funny one with the great sense of humor," "The smart one," "The creative one," "Tons of fun," "Ms. Enthusiasm," "Jolly fellow," "The lady with the sweet spirit." Do, any of these sound familiar?

In the process of defining ourselves, we developed some wonderful skills and very admirable qualities; and what extraordinary people we have become!

It has been my privilege to travel to meet so many of you, to get to know some of you and to share in your success and this remarkable transformation of who you were to finally who you are now! May I share with you a comment from a psychologist about his experience in working with some of our bariatric patients? He said that he has never met more caring, sensitive, thoughtful and kind people. We have fostered these traits for many years and now, (now that we are who we have become only now in "normal bodies") many are finding the world a kinder place to be. Some are finding that where there were once brick walls, open doors present themselves. What a thrill it is to participate in all that a healthy lifestyle has to offer. What a thrill it is to be noticed, recognized, respected and even applauded!

It's exciting, yes, but scary too. Underneath it all, we are who we have always been, though we look differently, and as a result, people respond to us differently. New opportunities and experiences abound. Sometimes we feel like, "Look out world!" We find ourselves being assertive, even aggressive, and sometimes even intimidating. We find ourselves stepping forward, leading instead of following and accomplishing things that many only dream of.

"Our deepest fear is not that we are inadequate. Our deepest fear is that we are powerful beyond measure. It is our light, not our darkness, which most frightens us. We ask ourselves, who am I to be wonderful, talented, gorgeous, fabulous? Actually, who are you not to be? You are a child of

God. You're playing small doesn't serve the world. There is nothing enlightening about shrinking so that other people will not feel insecure around you. We were born to manifest God's glory within us. It is in everyone. And as we let our own light shine, we automatically give others permission to do the same. As we are liberated from our own fears, our presence liberates others."

- Marianne Williamson

As you go forward and continue to build and strengthen your relationships with your family and friends, as you continue to progress in your work and your careers, as you serve in your churches and communities, know that I applaud your success, and encourage you to "be all you can be." Be proud of who you are and be proud of the road you took to get here.

Now what?

"When you wish upon a star…

Makes no difference who you are
    [Or how much you weigh]

For when you wish upon a star
    [And are willing to take chances]

Your Dreams Come True!"

Next time you attend a support group meeting, take a moment to look around. Look to your left and to your right, look behind you and in front of you. The room will undoubtedly be filled with dreams come true; life-long dreams are coming true each day.

Recently, the American Society for Bariatric Surgery estimated that there were 45,000 bariatric surgeries performed in 2001 and estimated that 170,000 surgeries were performed in 2006. Thousands upon thousands of dreams are coming true.

Dreams are coming true each day: lifelong, unbelievable dreams. So what about your dreams? Are your dreams coming true? Have they already come true? And if so, are there more dreams? Do you have new dreams? Bigger dreams? If some of your dreams have come true, it is time to ask yourself, "Now what?"

The story of my dreams coming true truly catches people off guard. They are amazed when I share it with them. "Wow!" they say, "Dreams of this sort are nearly unheard of; very unique." But for the thousands reading this book, my successes are commonplace. I suspect that you have your own wonderful story to tell. I congratulate you for your success and encourage you to share your story with others. Great is the need for people who are willing to share their experiences to uplift, encourage and inspire others.

It has been my great pleasure through the years to learn of many successes, share in the dreams of literally thousands of weight-loss surgery patients. Some are common stories; others are extraordinary, like the following stories of three remarkable people who have touched my life, people whose great faith, commitment and hard work are an example to all of us.

SUE'S STORY

In March of 1995 Sue Pugmire found herself at the age of 34 weighing 540 pounds. She was unemployed, unhealthy, and very unhappy. She had just been fired from her job and forced to move from her apartment. She lived for six weeks in her brown 1986 Dodge Omni with all of her belongings and her cat, Klondyke. She recalls not caring anymore about much of anything. Dreams she had once had didn't seem at all possible now. She didn't care if she ever worked again, she didn't care about where she lived or even if she lived.

With the loving attention of dear friends and family members, she was encouraged to move to Salt Lake City to live with her mother. She worked a number of temporary jobs, trying desperately to pull her life together. Her weight, however, continued to escalate and her health deteriorated. In January of 1996, paramedics took her in an ambulance to the hospital in respiratory failure. After several days in ICU she was told she would not live more than three or four months unless she did something about her weight. With prayers, faith and encouragement from family and friends, Sue realized that "God had something in mind for her" and she decided then that she would do whatever it took to live.

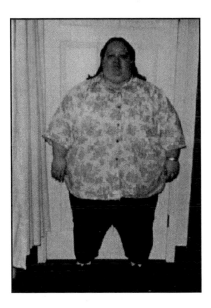

She was referred to Dr. Sherman Smith and had weight-loss surgery on April 5, 1996 – Good Friday. She recalls not waking up until Sunday, which, ironically, was Easter Morning. That had great significance to her as she began her new life that day, and she also began her renewed walk with the Lord.

During the weeks and months that followed, she struggled with her health and recovery, but during that time she found a great inner peace and re-committed herself to fulfilling a dream that had been long lost and forgotten. You see, at a mission conference in 1978, she felt "called" or inspired that she was to work with the youth of her church. And now, perhaps…perhaps that would be possible.

By the spring of 1997, one year later, Sue had lost 210 pounds. Her total weight loss today is 330 pounds.

Today she is living her dreams. She loves softball and not only does she play on a women's team but she recently coached a girl's fast-pitch softball team. And then there is golf, one of her life's passions. These days when she isn't working at LifeWay Christian Bookstore, you will find her playing golf.

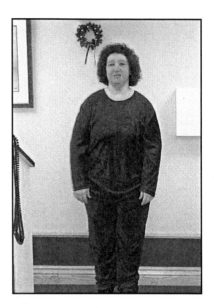

And as for dreams coming true, Sue was awarded her local minister's license and is well on her way to being ordained a Children's Minister in the First Church of the Nazarene. You see, her weight-loss was just the beginning. Sue took care of her weight problem and then asked herself, "Now what?"

BRIAN'S STORY

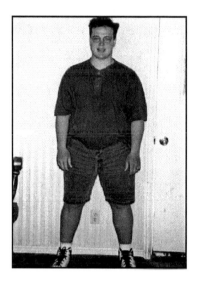

When you weigh 150 pounds in elementary school, you get made fun of. A lot. Though he was a happy, outgoing child on the inside, he was always depressed about his weight. His weight escalated through the years as he gained and gained and by the time he reached high school he weighed 245 pounds. He stayed pretty healthy and active. He played defense tackle for the Northridge High School football team, as well as shot put and discuss throw for the track team. He recalls carrying his weight well, though having a big belly really bothered him. He had a lot of friends, but never, ever dated. Girls, he said would kind of look the other way. He was afraid to ask anyone out for fear of rejection. Brian had friends, but no romance.

During his senior year, he injured his knees, and was down flat on his back for over three months. During those months his weight climbed to 305 pounds.

Since he was six years old, he dreamed of becoming a body builder, like his idol, Arnold Swartzenager. His dream seemed so out of reach, even unachievable, but it remained in the back of his mind. Someday . . . someday.

With the encouragement and support of his mother, a weight-loss surgery patient, he decided to have surgery on April 1, 1997. And within five months, Brian lost 105 pounds. His dreams of being a body builder were rekindled once again, and he started biking and weight lift-ing.

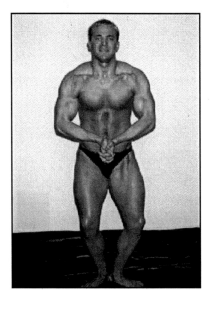

In February 1998 Brian was feeling healthy enough to serve a mission for his church, but it was cut short due to an illness. He returned home and had surgery to remove his gallbladder and repair a hernia. He lost 20 more pounds and was very sick. At 175 pounds, he decided that was it! He was going to be healthy and going to get the body he had always dreamed of. He began working out six days per week and dedicated himself to getting into better shape.

With determination and hard work, Brian trained in the gym five hours per day. On April 21, 1999, he competed for Mr. Utah Natural. In front of eight judges and an audience of 3,000, he went after a dream, and he placed fourth in the heavy-weight novice class.

Brian now has plans to compete again in the same pageant next April and go on to compete for thc Mr. Utah Cup. He lost his excess weight, and then asked himself, "Now what?"

BETTY'S STORY

If anyone asked, she wasn't much interested in getting married; after all, her career was the most important thing on her mind. With a degree in Journalism and Public Relations from the University of Oklahoma, Betty accepted a position with GE Capital Finance. Well, not exactly what she wanted, but it was a career nevertheless. She was confident and talented, but very unhappy. Her true desires-her secret dreams-included a husband, a family and a home. But she had resigned herself to believe that she would be big and alone forever and that would just have to be okay.

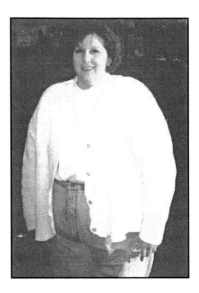

Weight was a battle she fought her entire life. With dozens of weight losses and gains through the years, depression and self-doubt became an additional challenge. And then came more depression and more doubt. Tired of failing and tired of waiting for the next "miracle drug," she knew she had to do something drastic. At 330 pounds with nothing to lose but weight and an entire life to gain, she had weight loss surgery in September of 1998.

As her excess weight came off, she began enjoying herself, enjoying just being herself, and enjoying the feeling of being well and healthy. She began thinking to herself that maybe, just maybe, it's not too late to have the dreams of her heart.

With her experience in corporate strategic planning, Betty decided to do a little life planning. On a business trip in a hotel room, she mapped out her goals and dreams with butcher paper on all the walls and Post-It notes everywhere. She rekindled her dreams and set her goals. In addition to the little goals, she added what seemed the most momentous: to marry, have a family, and start her own business.

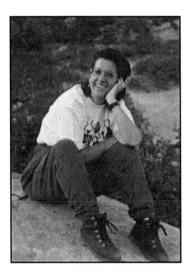

So, she began to do those things that she had always wanted to do: hiking, biking, dating and scuba diving. In May of 1999, she met her knight in shining armor: a loving, caring, respectful man with a heart of gold who treats her like royalty. In July of 2002, with all dreams in common, they began their new life together and she became his princess bride.

And as if that wasn't enough, Betty went on to fulfill another of her life's goals. She recently quit her job of 13 years and began a business of her own. She, too, saw her weight loss as a new beginning. She took care of her weight problem and then asked herself, "Now what?"

Each of these people used their weight-loss as a spring-board to their future, as the catalyst for change and as a new beginning. Having been blessed with healthier, normal bodies, they said to themselves, "Now what?!" I too, have seen my dreams come true and continue to say to myself, "Now what?"

Now, may I pose that all-important question to each of you: "Now what??" What wonderful and fulfilling things await you? What new dreams might you dream? And where will you go from here? And who might be there to help you?

Have you ever felt that while you're tying balloons to your lawn chair there was someone right behind you tying bricks to your feet? Do you have people in your life like that? People that are keeping you grounded, keeping you here, keeping you safe, keeping you from reaching, from trying and doing. I suspect that you have identified one if not more than one person in your mind. Now ask yourself why? Why do they do that? What are they afraid of? What are these people afraid of? What is it that motivates them to keep you down? No doubt, there are different reasons for different people. Perhaps they are afraid that you will suc-ceed leaving them behind?

I remember wanting to skydive in high school; I took les-sons and everything, learned the ripcord thing, and I was ready to go. My mom said, "You know, it is really warming up, I think it will be better if you wait until it kind of cools off in the Fall." And then Fall came around and she said, "It is getting awfully chilly I think we should wait until Spring." And she talked me out of it. Because she didn't want me to get hurt. There are people like that in our lives. They are important. We love them, they care very much about our well-being. Some of them are worried about our success and the effect it will have on their own place in our world if we choose to change. Whatever the reason, there will always be people in our lives, who do all they can to try to keep us the same.

Through the years I have come to realize how important is it to surround myself with people who understand why I do what I do. People who understand what it is that drives me. You too, must find people in your life who have a belief in you; people who understand your spirit and your far-reaching goals and dreams and ideas. The following story illustrates this point beautifully.

A young mother wanted to have her little boy learn to play the piano. He was taking lessons and she was just sure that he had all the makings of a famous pianist. With that in mind, she made arrangements for the two of them to go to Carnegie Hall to the see the master, Ignacy Paderewsky, play. And so she dressed her son up in his little suit and took him to the concert. They found their seats, settled down real close to the stage. As they did, the mother turned around and noticed one of her friends nearby and they started chatting. When the mother turned back around the little boy was gone, and she panicked immediately. Where had he gone? Where did he go? Oh, no!

Moments later, she noticed her son up on the stage, at the grand piano in Carnegie Hall, playing chop sticks. He was just learning the little chop sticks piece, and the audience was aghast, "Somebody stop him!" "That is awful!" "That is terrible!" "How embarrassing!" "Somebody get him down from there!" "Who would bring a child to this?" "What a disgrace!" From the back of the room came the master, Ignacy Paderewsky at a dead run, down through the audience, through the aisle, up onto the stage, around behind the little boy. He began playing an accompanying melody to the little boy's chop sticks and as he did, he gently encouraged, saying, "Don't stop, keep going, you're doing fine, don't stop, keep going, you're doing fine."

How often in our lives do we feel like we are playing chop sticks at Carnegie Hall? We need people to surround us that say with sincerity, "You're doing great, don't stop, keep going, you're doing fine."

As we are running our race, we need people at the sidelines saying, "You were not meant for failure here, get up and win that race."

The simple fact that you're reading this book shows that you want to learn and grow and take responsibility for your life and your success. You must surround yourself with people who know why these kinds of things are important to you. Surround yourself with winners. Learn of them. Learn from them and be uplifted and inspired by them.

Paying It Forward

The Bridge Builder

An old man going a long highway
Came at the evening, cold and gray,
To a chasm vast and wide and steep,
With water rolling cold and deep.
The old man crossed in the twilight dim
The sullen stream had no fears for him;
But he turned when safe on the other side,
And built a bridge to span the tide.
"Old man," said a fellow pilgrim near,
"You are wasting your strength with building here.
Your journey will end with the ending day,
You never again will pass this way.
You've crossed the chasm, deep and wide,
Why build you this bridge at eventide?"
The builder lifted his old gray head.
"Good friend, in the path I have come," he said,
"There followeth after me today
A youth whose feet must pass this way.
The chasm that was as nought to me
To that fair-haired youth may a pitfall be;
He, too, must cross in twilight dim—
Good friend, I am building this bridge for him."
--Will Allen Dromgoole

It is so very important that we, as today's weight-loss surgery patients, recognize and are grateful to courageous souls who opted to have weight loss surgery when it wasn't the "in thing" to do–those daring few from the late 70's and early 80's who experienced both successes and failures and in doing so have provided us with greater understanding of what it takes to make the surgical treatment of obesity our answer. Has someone led the way for you, inspired you, encouraged you? Often weight-loss surgery patients express heartfelt gratitude, not only to their surgeons for having saved their life, but to friends and family members, neighbors, work associates and even strangers who have motivated them and provided them with the encouragement and support they needed to move forward on their journey.

To those looking for a way to express their gratitude, may I encourage you to turn and help others along their way. Become involved; lead a support group; become a volunteer; serve on a patient committee; lobby for better insurance coverage for weight-loss surgery; help new or struggling patients with online posts of encouragement and support. Give back by paying it forward.

Service is the rent we pay to live on this planet. We have all warmed ourselves by fires we did not build. And drunk from wells we did not dig. We must now, dig more wells and build more fires. – Nido Qubein

Willie's Story

It was a long drive for Willie Collins only to find that his trip to see a bariatric surgeon in Houston, Texas was for naught.

After a short consultation the surgeon told him, "No one can touch you, you are just TOO big! No one will be able to keep you breathing on the table. I don't think your wife wants to bring you all the way to Houston and then go home a widow."

The challenge that Willie faced, back in the spring of 1978, is one that many super-morbidly obese patients have had to deal with. Desperately needing a surgical treatment for their obesity, but thought by many to be too great a risk. And to make the likelihood of treatment even more challenging, most bariatric surgeons and hospitals are simply not equipped to handle patients over 500 pounds.

Willie, weighing in on truck scales at 768 pounds, had only one possible option. He was told, that if he were to go home and lose 200-300 pounds, then he could return for surgery. He did return home, but there he continued his search for someone, somewhere, who would provide him what he felt was his only option, life-saving bariatric surgery.

Both of Willie's parents were heavy and delt with many co-morbidities relating to their weight. They both died, in their late 60's. Not wanting to share in their fate, Willie did all he could to stay healthy and has done his best to enjoy

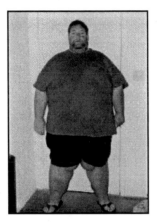

an active life. He has always been athletic, playing high school football and participating in family activities and sports with his children. Though his blood pressure and cholesterol levels were normal, his size made it difficult to function. A plant operator, Willie was placed on disability and was forced to leave his employment.

Willie turned to the West to one of the nation's renowned bariatric surgeons, Dr. Mal Fobi. Willie, was the largest person ever to undergo weight loss surgery, weighing in on truck scales, he had the Fobi Pouch operation on May 13th, 1998.

Against all odds, Willie survived that surgery, but his adventure had just begun. He returned home from the hospital one week later and thanks his wonderful friend, Jerry, also a patient, for his encouragement and support before and during his recovery. He was my mentor," Willie states, "And I am forever grateful."

More surgeries followed. Within eighteen months, Willie lost down to 430 pounds! And then his weight loss stopped. (I understand this is common among those with so much weight to lose). Dr. Fobi followed Willie's initial operation with a distal Roux-en-Y revision surgery and then some plastic surgery to remove Willie's excess skin on his breast, stomach, arms and thighs. 2003 found Willie a happy and healthy, six foot three, 255 pound, 45 year old.

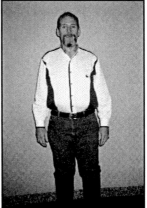

Willie committed his life to educating, supporting and encouraging others along their way. Willie has shared his miraculous story with thousands and no doubt has inspired many who thought their case hopeless.

It is with great sadness that I share with you the news of Willie's passing. In November of 2005, just two years after the publication of his story in this book, Willie died from complications resulting from a bowel obstruction. His wonderful spirit of love and genuine care for his fellow WLS patients will live in our hearts forever. May each of us follow his example by paying it forward to those who are struggling with the effects of the disease of obesity.

Tammy's Story - Duodenal Switch

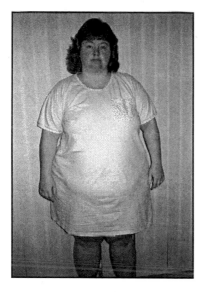

As a teenager, I participated in all the fad diets along with the rest of my size 8 girlfriends because that's what teenage girls do, right? I lived on Diet Coke, Peppermint Certs, and Trident gum and ate only one meal each day to achieve my biggest goal…fitting into my boyfriends Levis (size 29)!

I didn't really struggle with the issues of real obesity until I started having children. I never quite got rid of that last few pounds after the first baby and then added about 20 more after the second. I was in an unhappy marriage for several years and my weight continued to creep upward until I reached a new high of 240 pounds. It knew it was time to make some changes for myself and I divorced my husband. I began to feel better about myself, regained my self confidence and self esteem and lost 70 pounds. A few years later, I remarried and after the birth of my third child, my weight began to increase again. After struggling for over seven years on my own, I decided to research bariatric surgery. I decided that the Duodenal Switch was the right surgery for me, even though there was a 6 month wait for my surgeon, Dr. Henry Buchwald.

While I waited, I had to 'convince' my husband and that was not an easy task. In fact, it was not possible. He believed that I just needed to "try harder" and that I hadn't "exhausted all of my options" yet. I started the Atkins® diet and began to lose weight. I heard a lot of, "I told you so" but, I tried to ignore them and I really hoped this time the weight would stay off and, as much as I hated to admit it, maybe my husband was right. I cancelled my duodenal switch surgery date for Dec. 2002 because I lost 85 pounds on Atkins®. It was the most success I ever had with a single diet. However, in Feb. 2003, I required treatment at the Mayo Clinic for slow colonic transit and was asked to stop the diet by my doctors. I did, and then rapidly began to regain weight.

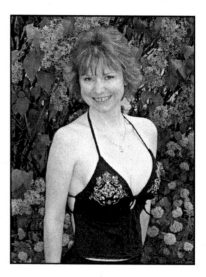

By July 2003, I was well on my way to having regained everything I had lost and probably more. I scoured the internet and printed out everything I could find regarding the favorable outcomes obtained by duodenal switch patients and placed it on the table in front of my husband. I wasn't asking for his permission at that point, I just wanted him to be well informed, because I was moving forward. By the time my surgery day came, my husband was on board and very supportive.

On the morning of surgery, I weighed 285 pounds. My duodenal switch surgery was preformed as an open procedure and after 5 days in the hospital, I returned home and had a completely uneventful recovery. I have lost all of my excess weight with absolutely no weight regain. I wore a bikini for the first time in my life the week I turned 40 years old. I have gone from size 26 to size 2. My pre-op BMI was 48.9 and now is a healthy 20.8.

"I have lost 164 pounds and in the process, have gained more self-worth and self-esteem than I've ever had in my life."

I had the wonderful opportunity of meeting Tammy at a WLS conference in 2005.

I was not only impressed with her success, but inspired by her wonderful energy and her commitment to become a well educated advocate for DS patients.

Tammy leads local and online DS support groups, is writing a handbook for duodenal switch patients, volunteers at local hospitals, and assists with insurance appeals. She leads by example and has dedicated her life to giving back by paying it forward.

Janean Hall

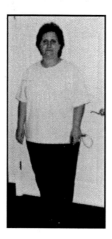

Janean Hall is an admired WLS patient and respected Bariatric professional, known for her heartfelt dedication & commitment to weight loss surgery patients throughout the world. A weight loss surgery patient from 1997, Janean has been an exemplary patient maintaining a loss of over 135 pounds. She credits much of her success to her commitment to a lifetime of living the Success Habits Principles.

Janean's personal experience, coupled with the insight she has gained through the years working with literally thousands of weight-loss surgery patients, makes her a rare asset to the Bariatric community.

Her contributions have been many including: The creation & development of a comprehensive dietary guidelines book and supplementary resources, multiple patient classes & programs and her most recent work has been the creation of a 5-day kick start food plan for patients who are stuck on a plateau or are needing to get back on track. She is the author of the Kick Start and Maintenance Mentality books, and is pursuing certification as a Bariatric Life Coach through Bariatric University.

Janean is one of the partners of Bariatric Support Centers International, is a National Trainer for BSCI's Support Group Leader Training & Back On Track Facilitator programs. Janean is the creative mind behind the development of the Success Habits Lesson kits now being used in hundreds of support groups throughout the country.

Whether in one on one counseling, teaching in a classroom setting, or presenting a training workshop, participants learn from Janean's wisdom, are motivated by her example and inspired by her heart.

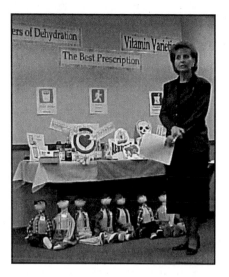

I am delighted to introduce you to this remarkable woman who has been an inspiration and support to me for many years. This single mother of 6 children and grandmother of 14, is the finest example of paying it forward that I have ever had the privilege of knowing. May we all continue to be motivated by her example.

Aspiring Higher

The Success Habits™ principles I have shared with you throughout this book, are essential to long term weight control for weight-loss surgery patients. As you can see from the stories shared, these principles work regardless of the type of procedure you select. My staff and I are working diligently to continue our research and understanding of these important principles. I hope that this overview has been enlightening and has motivated you to seriously consider implementing them into your life. In doing so, I am confident that you will reach and maintain your goals.

Through the years I have been blessed to have had the wonderful privilege of speaking to many groups of bariatric surgery patients throughout the country. I have been a featured speaker at support group meetings, patient conferences, patient reunions and fashion shows, even on several "Celebrating Success" cruises. My message has always been the same; and as I close this book with this chapter, may I leave you with that same message of the importance of aspiring higher. May you recognize that you are a truly remarkable individual. This is evidenced by the fact that you were willing to take responsibility for where you were and take action to do whatever it took to improve your

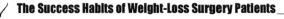

health. You have unique talents, skills and experiences. You have abilities that you have spent a lifetime perfecting and now, you are blessed to have all that you are and all that you know, inside a "normal" body.

> "So tell us what of happiness, how do we become happy?" And he simply replied, "If you want to be happy, then be happy."

In addition to being grateful for this wonderful gift of a thinner, healthier body, may I encourage you to actually do something with it? Do something extraordinary, something that will matter to others, something that will improve the quality of life for another. In this closing chapter, I am going to share with you some things from my head and some things from my heart. I hope that you have found something that will positively impact your life and will feel that your time reading this book has been time well spent. May each of your days from now on be well spent. May you learn to choose, each day, to be happy.

A man by the name of Joseph Smith said, "Happiness is the object and design of our existence."

An Indian guru was once asked, "So tell us what of happiness, how do we become happy?" And he replied simply, "If you want to be happy, then BE happy."

My grandmother passed away at the young age of 65. For

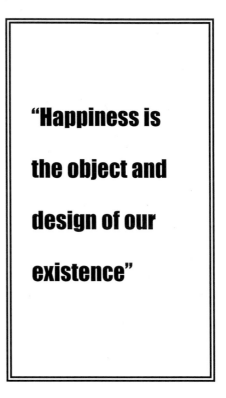

"Happiness is the object and design of our existence"

twenty years of her life she lived with a very serious heart condition. She had a number of open-heart surgeries and month after month and year after year she was told that time was about up. "We don't know how long you have left, but we can't do anything more for you. We think you know that your heart is going to give out soon. We are just sorry we can't tell you when. Day after day, and week after week, and year after year she lived with the understanding that her time was just about up, that tomorrow might be it.

Watching her, I began to realize what was truly important in life. My grandmother read, studied, and learned, she was very quick to forgive people and always surrounded herself with family.

It would be foolish of us to wait until our days are numbered to really take responsibility for where our lives ought to be, could be and should be. We need to be happy now by simply choosing to be happy.

Will Rogers said, "I want to live until I die."

George Burns, you will remember, lived to be 101. I saw a television interview he participated in when he turned 100 years old. The interviewer asked, "Well, George, look at you, you are just fit as a fiddle and doing well at 100, but tell me, how many of those cigars do you smoke each day?" George said, "Well, I don't know, five or six." And the reporter replied, "Oh, really? Well, how many of those martini's do you drink?" George said, "I don't know, maybe six or seven." And the reporter asked, "So what does your doctor say about that?" George replied, "Don't know, he's dead."

Here is a quote from Jorge Luis Borges as he was nearing the end of his life:

"If I had my life to live over, I would try to make more mistakes next time. I would relax. I would limber up. I would be crazier than I've been on this trip. I know very few things I'd take seriously any more. I'd certainly be less hygienic. I would take more chances, I would take more trips, I would scale more mountains, I would swim more rivers, and I would watch more sunsets. I would eat more ice cream and fewer beans. I would have more actual troubles and fewer imaginary ones. Oh, I've had my moments, and if I had it to do all over again, I'd have many more of them, in fact I'd try not to have anything else, just moments, one after another, instead of living so many years ahead of my day. If I had it to do all over again, I'd travel lighter, much lighter than I have. I would start barefoot earlier in the spring, and I'd stay that way much later in the fall. And I would ride more merry-go-rounds, and catch more gold rings, and greet people and pick more flowers and dance more often. If I had it to do all over again–but you see, I don't."

What great counsel.

A MOMENT IN TIME

This was a moment in time I will never forget, and in it I learned a very valuable life lesson from a new friend of mine, Wayne Bonner. Wayne is a very reserved, calm, mild-mannered, 18-year-old. I have an 18-year-old son and I said to him one day, "You know, that Wayne Bonner is kind of a nice kid." And my son replied, "Yeah, he is a pretty nice kid, but you ought to see him wake board. I thought, "Wake board? That's a pretty extreme sport, especially for such a mild-mannered kid." Let me tell you what wake boarding is. A wake board is about two feet wide and about four feet long. The rider is anchored to the top of the board with boots and is dragged behind a boat in a manner similar to that of a water skier. My family water skis, we sled, we do air chairs, and tubing, but the thing teenagers love the most is wake boarding.

You start out with the wake board parallel to the back of the boat as you're floating in the water, facing the ski boat. As the boat picks up speed, you're pulled out of the water and must then turn the board so it is facing the ski boat and you're riding it like a surf board. The first thing a wake boarder has to learn is to get out of the water and up on top of the board. The second thing they learn is to be able to move back and forth from side to side; going back and forth over the boat wake. Next, they learn how to "catch air." Catching air means you can see air between the bottom of the wake board and the water. On our boat we have what is called a tower, which holds the rope way up high so the wake boarder can get more maneuverability. The wake boarder starts on one side of the wake, hits the wake and catches air. The trick is to land safely on the other side of the wake.

So Wayne Bonner is apparently a fabulous wake boarder. One summer day we took a group of teenagers out on an excursion and we were all having a wonderful time. Wayne Bonner was there with his family and their really cool boat. And I thought, "Oh, wow, I get to watch him." He was absolutely phenomenal. He was doing what is called a "grab," which means that he would jump up and grab the bottom of the board and pull it up so he would catch even more air. It looked really great.

At lunchtime Wayne said to my husband and I, "You know, I would like to go on your boat with the tower." I thought, "Cool! Wayne Bonner is going to go on our boat! And so we were going along and he was doing all these grabs and jumps. And we were so cool; we had Wayne Bonner with us. I wanted to say, "Look at us!" After a while my husband steered the boat toward a narrow channel. On one side of the channel were four or five ski boats all tied together facing the same direction, with a couple of kids playing in the water. Twenty or thirty people were walking back and forth along the backs of the boats; we called it a party barge. On the other side of the channel was the shoreline where people were playing volleyball, sun bathing, playing in the water, picnicking, and just having a good time. I thought, "Oh, we're going to go right between all these people. I wonder what Wayne will do!"

Wayne saw where we were going and he went over as far as he could to one side and raised his hand high up in the air to get everyone's attention. And I thought, "Oh, my goodness, I wonder what he is going to do. I hope it's good because now everyone is watching." Wayne had everyone's attention. He took off like a shot from the left side, hit the wake, did a complete somersault in the air, and landed on the right side of the wake. Upon completion of this phenomenal stunt, Wayne immediately raised his spare hand and waved to the left and waived to the right. Needless to say, the crowds went wild. It was unbelievable, oh they were just clapping and screaming and cheering. And I was just amazed. It was incredible. It was perfect – an absolutely perfect moment in time for this young man. It was beautiful and inspiring to watch.

Everybody was watching, and as he prepared to climb back into the boat everyone was still clapping and kids were saying, "Wow, Wayne, you rock!" We were all so excited for him. As he got into the boat, I said, "Oh Wayne, I have got to tell you that was absolutely phenomenal. I couldn't believe it. You were so fantastic." And I enthusiastically started to recount to him what we saw: "You went over to the side of the boat and you raised your hand up..." And then he stopped me. And then came the lesson of a lifetime. He said, "When I did that, I *had* to land it."

At that moment in time, when this young man raised his hand high above his head, in his mind, there was no more doubt, there were no more questions, there was no more fear. His decision was made then and there; all that was left was the actual jump.

You have made an important, life-changing decision. Going "under the knife" for weight-loss surgery was not an easy decision to make. But, you made it anyway. Along with that decision must come your firm and unwavering commitment to follow through. I have shared with you experiences, stories, ideas, and challenges to teach you the Success Habits™ principles. May you understand them, internalize them and make them part of your commitment to a lifetime of good health and weight maintenance.

Just like Wayne Bonner did, I encourage you to make that commitment right here, right now. As you do so, may you recognize your extraordinary potential and may you use this wonderful gift of health to dream bigger dreams, reach further and aspire higher!

Yours for Greater Health and Happiness,

Colleen

Bibliography

Andrews, Gaye, PhD, MFCC (1997) "Intimate Saboteurs", *Obesity Surgery,* Vol 7, Rapid Science Publishers 445-448

Bartz, Tammy, (2005) *Strength-n-Sculpt* Bariatric Support Centers International

Carroll, Lewis (1872) *Through the Looking Glass*

Cook, Colleen M. (2003) Final Success Workbook, Bariatric Support Centers International

Cook, Colleen M., (2005) Goal Getting, Bariatric Support Centers International

Cook, CM; Edwards, Charles B. MD, (1999) "The Success Habits of Long-Term Gastric Bypass Patients", *Obesity Surgery*, Vol 9, No1, February 1999, Lippincott-Raven Publishers, USA

Flanagan, Laytham, MD, (1996) "Measurement of the Functional Pouch Volume Following Gastric Bypass Procedure", *Obesity Surgery*, 38-43

Fulghum, R. (1986) *All I Really Need To Know I Learned in Kindergarten*, Ivy Books, New York

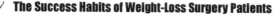
Hall, Janean G., (2005) *Maintenance Mentality* Bariatric Support Centers International

Hall, Janean G., Kenneth A. Miller, (2005) *How To Kick Start Your Weight Loss* Bariatric Support Centers International

Jacques, Jacqueline, ND, (2006) *Micronutrition for the Weight loss Surgery Patient*

Miller, Kenneth A., (2005) *Exchanging Habits*, Bariatric Support Centers International

Smith, Hyrum W., (1995) *The 10 Natural Laws of Successful Time and Life Management*, Warner Books

Williams, Margery (1987) *The Velveteen Rabbit*, Ideals Publishing Corp.

Footnotes

1. Fairfield KM, Fletcher RH. Vitamins for chronic disease prevention in adults: scientific review. JAMA 2002; 287:3116-3126.

2. Avinoah E, Ovnat A, Charuzi I. Nutritional status seven years after Roux-en-Y weight-loss surgery surgery. Surgery 1992 Feb;111(2):137-42.

3. Srinivasan VS. Bioavailability of nutrients. J Nutr 2001 Apr;131(4 Suppl):1349S-50S.

4. Brolin RE, Leung M. Survey of vitamin and mineral supplementation after weight-loss surgery and biliopancreatic diversion for morbid obesity. Obesity Surgery 1999 Apr;9(2):150-4.

Appendix A

Helpful People, Programs & Products

BARIATRIC ASSOCIATIONS
American Society for Bariatric Surgery
7328 West University Avenue, Suite F
Gainesville, FL 32607
www.asbs.org

Obesity Action Coalition
Jo Nadglowski, President, CEO
www.obesityaction.org

BARIATRIC EVENTS
www.bariatricsupportcenter.com
www.bariatricspeakers.com

BARIATRIC LIFE COACHING
Bariatric University
www.bariatricsupportcenter.com
www.bariatricu.com

BARIATRIC SUPPORT
BSCI Dream Team
www.bariatricsupportcenter.com

BARIATRIC NEWSLETTERS & JOURNALS

Bariatric Times
Professional Peer Reviewed Publication
www.bariatrictimes.com

Bariatrics Today
WLS Practice Management
www.bariatricstoday.com

Beyond Change Newsletter
Jacquelyn Smiertka, RN Editor
www.beyondchange-obesity.com

O H Magazine
Obesity Help
www.obesityhelp.com

Obesity Surgery Journal
Mervyn Deitel, Editor
www.obesitysurgery.com

WLS Lifestyles Magazine
Dan Babbino, Rebecca Riccard
www.wlslifestyles.com

BSCI eNewsletter
Bariatric Support Centers International
www.bariatricsupportcenter.com

BARIATRIC DISCOUNT PRODUCTS
www.barisaver.com

BMI CALCULATOR
Bariatric Support Centers International
4001 South 700 East, Suite 40
Salt Lake City, UT 84107
www.bariatricsupportcenter.com

DAILY RECORD OF ACCOUNTABILITY
Bariatric Support Centers International
www.bariatricsupportcenter.com

LEGAL COUNSEL
Obesity Law and Advocacy Center, Walter Lindstrom
www.obesitylaw.com

SUPPORT GROUPS
International Support Group Registry
www.bariatricsupportgroups.com

Support Group Leader Training
www.bariatricsupportcenter.com

Support Group Leader Resources
www.bariatricsupportcenter.com

VITAMINS AND SUPPLEMENTS
Bariatric Advantage
www.bariatricadvantage.com
www.barisaver.com

WEIGHT GAIN
Back On Track Programs & Resources
www.bariatricsupportcenter.com
Toll free: 800-339-9129

Record of Progress- Weight-loss Chart
www.bariatricsupportcenter.com
Toll free: 800-339-9129

Protein/Vegetable Recipes
www.bariatricsupportcenter.com
Toll free: 800-339-9129
www.chefdave.org

Appendix B

Body Mass Index Chart

Determining Your Body Mass Index (BMI)

BARIATRIC SUPPORT CENTERS
INTERNATIONAL

KEY

Underweight:	< 19
Normal	20 - 24
Overweight	25 - 29
Obese	30 - 34
Severely Obese	35 - 39
Morbidly Obese	> 40

Equations

Body Mass Index = kg / m^2
1 lb = .45 kg
1 in = .0254 m

Bariatric Support Center
1160 E 3900 S - Suite 4200
Salt Lake City, UT 84124
801-268-6262
Fax: 801-268-6168
1-800-339-9129
www.bariatricsupportcenter.com

Height (Feet and Inches)

Weight (Pounds)	5'0"	5'1"	5'2"	5'3"	5'4"	5'5"	5'6"	5'7"	5'8"	5'9"	5'10"	5'11"	6'0"	6'1"	6'2"	6'3"	6'4"
100	20	19	18	18	17	17	16	16	15	15	14	14	14	13	13	12	12
105	21	20	19	19	18	17	17	16	16	16	15	15	14	14	13	13	13
110	21	21	20	19	19	18	18	17	17	16	16	15	15	15	14	14	13
115	22	22	21	20	20	19	19	18	17	17	17	16	16	15	15	14	14
120	23	23	22	21	21	20	19	19	18	18	17	17	16	16	15	15	15
125	24	24	23	22	21	21	20	20	19	18	18	17	17	16	16	16	15
130	25	25	24	23	22	22	21	20	20	19	19	18	18	17	17	16	16
135	26	26	25	24	23	22	22	21	21	20	19	19	18	18	17	17	16
140	27	26	26	25	24	23	23	22	21	21	20	20	19	18	18	17	17
145	28	27	27	26	25	24	23	23	22	21	21	20	20	19	19	18	18
150	29	28	27	27	26	25	24	23	23	22	22	21	20	20	19	19	18
155	30	29	28	27	27	26	25	24	24	23	22	22	21	20	20	19	19
160	31	30	29	28	27	27	26	25	24	24	23	22	22	21	21	20	19
165	32	31	30	29	28	27	27	26	25	24	24	23	22	22	21	21	20
170	33	32	31	30	29	28	27	27	26	25	24	24	23	22	22	21	21
175	34	33	32	31	30	29	28	27	27	26	25	24	24	23	22	22	21
180	35	34	33	32	31	30	29	28	27	27	26	25	24	24	23	22	22
185	36	35	34	33	32	31	30	29	28	27	27	26	25	24	24	23	23
190	37	36	35	34	33	32	31	30	29	28	27	26	26	25	24	24	23
195	38	37	36	35	33	32	31	31	30	29	28	27	26	26	25	24	24
200	39	38	37	35	34	33	32	31	30	30	29	28	27	26	26	25	24
205	40	39	37	36	35	34	33	32	31	30	29	29	28	27	26	26	25
210	41	40	38	37	35	34	33	32	31	30	29	28	28	27	26	26	26
215	42	41	39	38	37	36	35	34	33	32	31	30	29	28	28	27	26
220	43	42	40	39	38	37	36	34	33	32	32	31	30	29	28	27	27
225	44	43	41	40	39	37	36	35	34	33	32	31	30	29	28	28	27
230	45	43	42	41	39	38	37	36	35	34	33	32	31	30	30	29	28
235	46	44	43	42	40	39	38	37	36	35	34	33	32	31	30	29	29
240	47	45	44	43	41	40	39	38	36	35	34	33	33	32	31	30	29
245	48	46	45	43	42	41	40	38	37	36	35	34	33	32	31	31	30
250	49	47	46	44	43	42	40	39	38	37	36	35	34	33	32	31	30
255	50	48	47	45	44	42	41	40	39	38	37	36	35	34	33	32	31
260	51	49	48	46	45	43	42	41	40	38	37	36	35	34	33	32	32
265	52	50	48	47	45	44	43	42	40	39	38	37	36	35	34	33	32
270	53	51	49	48	46	45	44	42	41	40	39	38	37	36	35	34	33
275	54	52	50	49	47	46	44	43	42	41	39	38	37	36	35	34	33
280	55	53	51	50	48	47	45	44	43	41	40	39	38	37	36	35	34
285	56	54	52	50	49	47	46	45	43	42	41	40	39	38	37	36	35
290	57	55	53	51	50	48	47	45	44	43	42	40	39	38	37	36	35
295	58	56	54	52	51	49	48	46	45	44	42	41	40	39	38	37	36
300	59	57	55	53	51	50	48	47	46	44	43	42	41	40	39	37	37
305	60	58	56	54	52	51	49	48	46	45	44	43	41	40	39	38	37
310	61	59	57	55	53	52	50	49	47	46	44	43	42	41	40	39	38
315	62	60	58	56	54	52	51	49	48	47	45	44	43	42	40	39	38
320	62	60	59	57	55	53	52	50	49	47	46	45	43	42	41	40	39
325	63	61	59	58	56	54	52	51	49	48	47	45	44	43	42	41	40
330	64	62	60	58	57	55	53	52	50	49	47	46	45	44	42	41	40
335	65	63	61	59	58	56	54	52	51	49	48	47	45	44	43	42	41
340	66	64	62	60	58	57	55	53	52	50	49	47	46	45	44	42	41
345	67	65	63	61	59	57	56	54	52	51	50	48	47	46	44	43	42
350	68	66	64	62	60	58	56	55	53	52	50	49	48	46	45	44	43
355	69	67	65	63	61	59	58	56	54	52	51	50	48	47	46	44	43
360	70	68	66	64	62	60	58	56	55	53	52	50	49	47	46	45	44
365	71	69	67	65	63	61	59	57	55	54	52	51	50	48	47	46	44
370	72	70	68	66	64	62	60	58	56	55	53	52	50	49	48	46	45
375	73	71	69	66	64	62	61	59	57	55	54	52	51	49	48	47	46
380	74	72	70	67	65	63	61	60	58	56	55	53	52	50	49	47	46
385	75	73	70	68	66	64	62	60	59	57	55	54	52	51	49	48	47
390	76	74	71	69	67	65	63	61	59	58	56	54	53	51	50	49	47
395	77	75	72	70	68	66	64	62	60	58	57	55	54	52	51	49	48
400	78	76	73	71	69	67	65	63	61	59	57	56	54	53	51	50	49

Appendix C

Weight-loss Progress Chart–Cook

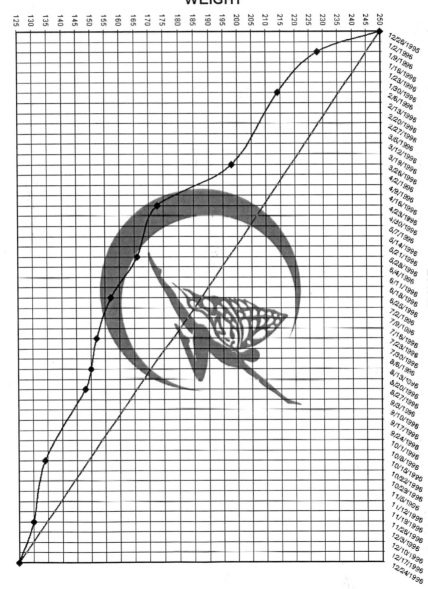

WEIGHT

DATE

Legend: —— Target Weight —+— Actual Weight

WEIGHT LOSS PROGRESS - COLLEEN COOK

For a customized weight loss progress chart, see www.bariatricsupportcenter.com

Appendix D

10-Year Weight-loss
Progress Chart–Cook

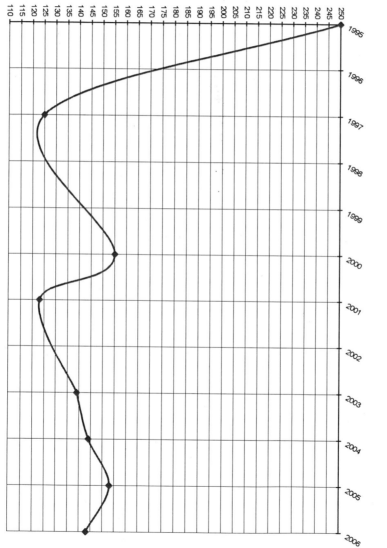

WEIGHT

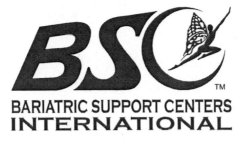

BARIATRIC SUPPORT CENTERS
INTERNATIONAL

MISSION STATEMENT

Our mission is to provide long-term educational and support resources for weight loss surgery patients and the professionals who serve them.

We assist people who struggle with the effects of the disease of obesity as they seek to improve their health and enhance the quality of their lives. Our programs, services and products are designed to meet the ever changing needs of bariatric patients. We provide quality support and educational resources for new, veteran, and struggling weight-loss surgery patients.

We assist bariatric professionals as they seek to improve the quality and consistency of their bariatric support and educational programs. Our professional training programs and resources are designed to support the people who support the patients. We provide valuable insight into the long-term needs of bariatric patients and provide the resources necessary to meet those needs.

BSCI GOVERNING VALUES

We are compassionate and understanding of those suffering from the disease of obesity.

We recognize and appreciate the intrinsic value of every human being and we are committed to assisting each individual person as they develop happy, healthy, productive lives and work to achieve their greatest potential.

We constantly strive to honor, respect and care for each individual member and associate while recognizing that our ability to help each individual can be no stronger than the health and strength of our business as a whole. Each of us desires to contribute more to the organization and society than we seek to take from them.

We believe in the importance of synergy and we seek to contribute our unique thoughts and experience to the collaborative efforts of staff members, volunteers and associates. We know that positive changes and improvements to our business and our lives comes through a spirit of cooperation.

We believe that everyone benefits as each of us exhibits an abundance mentality. We willingly share our knowledge, our resources, and our experience with others.

CONTACT INFORMATION

Bariatric Support Centers International
9257 South Redwood Road, Suite B
West Jordan, Utah 84088
Tel: (801) 327-6500 Fax: (801) 327-0600
www.bariatricsupportcenter.com
www.barisaver.com